Thriving with Kidney Disease

A Johns Hopkins Press Health Book

Thriving with
KIDNEY
DISEASE

A Practical Guide to Taking Care
of Your Kidneys and Yourself

2nd Edition

WALTER A. HUNT

Foreword by Ronald D. Perrone, MD

JOHNS HOPKINS UNIVERSITY PRESS

Baltimore

To my mother and sister, who did not survive kidney disease

———————

Note to the Reader: This book is not meant to substitute for medical care of people with kidney disease, and treatment should not be based solely on its contents. Instead, treatment must be developed in a dialogue between the individual and his or her physician. Our book has been written to help with that dialogue.

The author and publisher have made reasonable efforts to determine that the selection and dosage of drugs discussed in this text conform to the practices of the general medical community. The medications described do not necessarily have specific approval by the US Food and Drug Administration for use in the diseases and dosages for which they are recommended. In view of ongoing research, changes in governmental regulations, and the constant flow of information relating to drug therapy and drug reactions, the reader is urged to check the package insert of each drug for any change in indications and dosage and for warnings and precautions. This is particularly important when the recommended agent is a new and/or infrequently used drug.

Johns Hopkins University Press
2715 North Charles Street
Baltimore, Maryland 21218-4363
www.press.jhu.edu

Names: Hunt, W. A. (Walter A.) author.
Title: Thriving with kidney disease : a practical guide to taking care of your
    kidneys and yourself / Walter A. Hunt ; foreword by Ronald D. Perrone, MD.
Other titles: Kidney disease.
Description: Second edition. | Baltimore : Johns Hopkins University Press, 2022.
    | Series: A Johns Hopkins Press health book | Revision of: Kidney disease. c2011.
    | Includes bibliographical references and index.
Identifiers: LCCN 2021011717 | ISBN 9781421442891 (hardcover) |
    ISBN 9781421442907 (paperback) | ISBN 9781421442914 (ebook)
Subjects: LCSH: Kidneys—Diseases—Popular works.
Classification: LCC RC902 .H85 2022 | DDC 616.6/1—dc23
LC record available at https://lccn.loc.gov/2021011717

A catalog record for this book is available from the British Library.

Special discounts are available for bulk purchases of this book. For more information, please contact Special Sales at specialsales@jh.edu.

Contents

Foreword

Ronald D. Perrone, MD

It is a pleasure to write this foreword. Few books such as this one are available for those individuals diagnosed with kidney disease. Medical information about kidney disease and kidney failure is abundantly available, yet important perspectives from patients who have actually experienced kidney disease, kidney failure, and resulting dialysis and transplantation are not easily obtained. Walter Hunt has provided careful and easily understandable explanations for the layperson and offered his personal experience and perspective of the impact of kidney failure on his life. The revised second edition provides important updates, including coping skills for caregivers, kidney diseases in children, environmental causes of chronic kidney failure, conservative care for those who wish to decline treatment, gout, depression, sleep disturbances and depression in dialysis patients, and diet after transplantation. New approaches for potential treatments of chronic kidney disease, such as drug repurposing, gene editing, and biological markers, are also included.

I congratulate Dr. Hunt for providing this excellent guide for people with kidney disease!

I made the decision to enter the field of nephrology during my second year of medical school while doing my rotation on the inpatient nephrology service. Exposure to the miracle of transplantation and the lifesaving treatment of dialysis provided encouragement that I would have tools as a future physician to help patients overcome serious illness. Prior to the availability of these treatments, kidney failure was a disease with limited therapeutic options.

Working with newly diagnosed or long-term patients with kidney disease provides tremendous opportunities to intervene in their care. When I first encounter newly diagnosed patients with kidney disease, my hope for them is first to provide a diagnosis. If a treatment is available, I implement treatment to halt the inexorable progress of the disease. At this stage, it is very important to educate and inform them and their families about their disease and to enlist their participation in the patients' care. Finally, if necessary, I begin the prevention and management of potential complications and provide reassurance about the options for therapy, including dialysis and transplantation. This is not easily accomplished during a single visit but is the beginning of a long-term relationship with multiple opportunities for my patients to ask questions and to receive information from print or electronic sources that help them to understand and manage their disease.

Follow-up visits provide additional opportunities to reinforce the educational messages, to discuss compliance and participation in their care, to interact with additional family members, and to solidify the bond of comfort and trust that occurs with a long-term doctor-patient relationship. Different stages of the disease require different interventions. Long periods of stability are gratifying for all and don't necessarily require large amounts of discussion or intervention; however, by contrast, the approach of kidney failure and the need for dialysis or transplant can be anxiety provoking and requires frequent visits for education, counseling, and medication adjustment.

Receiving a diagnosis of kidney disease is frightening for most individuals. Vivid fears of dialysis and rapid progression to kidney failure are common. More often, interventions can slow the progression of chronic kidney disease and manage the complications. While these are not cures, as when an antibiotic cures pneumonia, nonetheless, these interventions can help to preserve health. Individuals with kidney disease should be fully engaged in the management of their disease as this offers the best possibility for slowing the progression and preventing complications. Being educated about the disease, being compliant with appropriate medication and diet, obtaining a home blood pressure device and regularly measuring/reporting their blood pressure, joining patient support groups, and supporting research and educational efforts by foundations such as the National Kidney Foundation or the Polycystic Kidney Disease Foundation can be empowering and provide multiple opportunities to improve their long-term outcome.

Dialysis is not a perfect treatment for kidney failure, but it saves lives and can provide a reasonable quality of life for those individuals who are compliant with their treatment and dietary and fluid restrictions. Improvements in dialysis technology and the increasing availability of home dialysis and daily dialysis treatments have greatly improved the outcomes for many individuals. Conservative management of advanced kidney failure has recently emerged as a viable option for those who wish to avoid dialysis, with a focus on quality not quantity of life. Transplantation, while not a cure for kidney disease, is an excellent treatment yet still requires frequent visits to medical providers, lots of pills, and potentially serious complications from these potent medications. Greatly improved quality of life and longer life result from this intervention, yet careful compliance and follow-up is still required.

As a physician who has not personally experienced kidney disease, my understanding of the terrifying nature of receiving a diagnosis of kidney disease has always been secondhand. *Thriving with Kidney Disease* provides an honest perspective from someone who has experienced loss of kidney function, received years of dialysis, and been successfully transplanted. These insights and personal experiences from the perspective of a patient and the easily understandable explanations of complicated biology and medical treatment are a tremendous resource. Further, the reassurance provided by someone who has already been there will hopefully provide some lessening of anxiety and fear for those who are newly diagnosed or are facing new treatments such as dialysis or transplantation. It is my hope that this book will provide guidance and companionship as you journey through the complexities of diagnosis and treatment of chronic kidney disease.

Preface

In the United States, over 786,000 people suffer from chronic kidney failure, requiring dialysis or transplantation. I am one of them. When my parents conceived me, I inherited a genetic defect that led to cysts forming in my kidneys, eventually destroying my kidney function. Called polycystic kidney disease, this genetic defect is the fourth leading cause of chronic kidney failure in the United States. I spent ten years dealing with it, including seven and a half years on dialysis with numerous complications, before receiving a successful kidney transplant.

When I first realized that my kidneys could fail, I searched for information that would help me prepare for what was to come. Plenty of information was available describing my disease and the ways in which doctors could treat chronic kidney failure. However, I could not find a systematic discussion of what it would be like to experience this disease and of how I would decide which treatment options would be best for me. I did not find my doctors particularly helpful. Although doctors might see patients dealing with chronic kidney failure all the time and have empathy for them, they might see the disease largely from a medical perspective but not necessarily from a personal one, since they had not experienced chronic kidney failure themselves.

Based on my experiences, I decided to write this book to fill the void for people like me who wanted practical information to help them navigate the whole process of understanding what causes chronic kidney failure, what patients can do to help themselves through this process, and what personal factors could help them in making decisions on their care. I believe that such information will help patients make better, more informed decisions, potentially leading to better outcomes, a sense of control over their conditions, and a better quality of life.

One advantage I have over many patients is my training and experience in medical research. Although I am not a physician, I could learn what I needed along the way to help me understand what was happening to me. Besides the medical aspects of my disease, I learned how to cope with many of the problems of chronic kidney failure. It is my sincere hope that this book will assist my fellow patients as they deal with their respective conditions.

In this new edition, I have updated the knowledge on what we know about the various causes of chronic kidney disease. In addition, I have added sections in several chapters to cover other topics not covered in the previous edition. For example, there are sections on coping skills for caregivers, kidney diseases in children, environmental causes of chronic kidney failure, conservative care for those who wish to decline treatment, gout, depression, sleep disturbances and depression in dialysis patients, and diet after transplantation. New approaches for potential treatment of chronic kidney disease include drug repurposing, gene editing, and biological markers.

In the chapters to follow, I have referenced publications on which the information provided is based, a list of which is provided toward the end of the book. I have included a list of organizations that can provide additional information and resources not specifically covered in this book. Because the meaning of some the scientific terms may be difficult to remember when used in other chapters, I have included a glossary that readers can consult without jumping to other parts of the book for definitions.

I want to give a special thanks to Dr. Ron Perrone at Tufts University in Boston, Massachusetts. Ron shared many hours of his time with me when I was developing the first edition, explaining kidney disease from a clinical perspective and ensuring that the information in this book was accurate. He did so with good cheer and thoroughly explained what I needed to know. Any inaccuracies that may have crept in after his thorough reviews and those of subsequent reviewers are my sole responsibility. I greatly appreciate Ron's time, scholarship, and collegial spirit in bringing this book to fruition.

In addition, I want to thank Johns Hopkins University Press for supporting this project, especially my editor, Joseph Rusko. His skill, support, and advice were indispensable in creating the final work. It was great working with him. I would also like to thank the skill of editors Michael Zieler and Andre Barnett in helping clarify the text and all others on the staff who helped make this book possible. I am grateful.

Finally, I feel eternal gratitude to the many health care professionals at Kaiser Permanente and Gambro (now DaVita) Healthcare, who kept me alive during the dark days of dialysis. Without them, I would have been dead years ago. I am very grateful to Dr. Nidhi Malik, my primary care physician, and Dr. Vasudha Narayana, my nephrologist, for their dedicated efforts on my behalf and for their rapid responses when I experienced many emergencies. I will never forget them.

I had a wonderful opportunity to participate in a clinical trial when I received my transplant. My experience enhanced my quality of life and reduced the likelihood of complications in the future. I extend my thanks to Drs. Allen Kirk, Douglas Hale, Rosalynn Mannon, and Monique Cho, as well as the staff in the transplant program at the National Institutes of Health for allowing me to participate in the trial. Above all, my heart goes out to the family of the 18-year-old boy who lost his life, so that I could live a better life. I can never repay that sacrifice.

Thriving with Kidney Disease

CHAPTER 1

Understanding Chronic Kidney Disease

O N AUGUST 11, 1997, a catheter was implanted in my abdomen so I could receive dialysis. My kidneys had failed. I could still urinate, but I couldn't eliminate all the waste products that I accumulated from food. It's natural to take urinating for granted— it's something we've done since the day we were born. As adults we think about going to the bathroom only when we can't get to one because we're trapped in a business meeting, say, or stuck in traffic. And we do not usually discuss urination in polite company. When we need to urinate, we just excuse ourselves or adopt a euphemism—we're going to the powder room or we're going to see a man about a horse.

When urinating is no longer a normal, almost trivial activity, our lives are altered. When urinating becomes a focus of our attention, our lives are radically changed. When my kidneys started to shut down, I found the prospect of kidney failure overwhelming. I had so many questions: *Why are my kidneys failing? Is there anything I can do to save my kidneys? How will I know when my kidneys have failed? What will it feel like when my kidneys fail? Is there a cure or treatment for kidney failure?*

The good news, as I found out, is that kidney failure is no longer a death sentence, as it once was. Those of us with kidney failure can still have productive lives. The bad news is that we may spend countless hours going to dialysis and doctors' offices and making sure we take all our medications. There are some aspects of the disease that we can't control. One aspect of the disease that we *can* control is how well we understand it. Understanding kidney failure—what causes it, how it may affect our lives, and what options we have—can help us take an active role in treating our disease, lifting our spirits, achieving a better outcome, and improving our quality of life.

How Many People Have It?

Chronic kidney disease (CKD) (chronic kidney disease, chronic kidney failure, and renal insufficiency are used interchangeably with CKD) can develop from many causes and results in a progressive decline in kidney function to the point of requiring treatment, such as dialysis (chapter 6) or transplantation (chapter 7). CKD proceeds in five stages over many years (chapter 4) and in the final stage is known as *kidney failure*, formerly known as end-stage renal disease.[1] Fortunately, not all cases of CKD progress to kidney failure. However, screening of those at risk is an important step.

CKD and especially kidney failure have been increasing rapidly worldwide over the past two decades, affecting almost one billion people and killing nearly one million, based on 2013 data,[2] and touching the lives of men more than women. Here is some insight into what the world has experienced.

The number of people with CKD (called *prevalence*) is not uniform throughout the world, and deaths from kidney failure are often higher in countries without enough facilities or financial resources for dialysis and transplantation. In other cases, significant minority populations tend to have higher prevalence rates of CKD than the majority population. Examples of the latter case are the United States, Canada, and Australia, whose minority populations show prevalence rates two to ten times higher than the majority population.

In general, the United States, Canada, East Asia, and Western Europe have the greatest problems with kidney failure, whereas much of Latin America, Southern Asia, and Eastern Europe have the fewest problems.[3] The major cause is diabetes. Kidney failure is seen more often in men than in women with only a few exceptions in minority populations. Although some regions of the world have an extremely higher problem with kidney failure than others do, the reasons for this are not yet understood, although it may have to do with diet (chapter 5). For more information about global prevalence and incidence of kidney failure, see the appendix.

With this brief global perspective of kidney disease, let us examine the data for the United States in more detail, since they are better characterized than the rest of the world and are more recent.[3] The total numbers of people with kidney failure and of new cases are among the highest in the world, although the number of people with CKD has been stabilizing over the past few years. Still, 15 percent of the population has CKD. By the end of 2018, over 786,000 people in the United States were being treated for kidney failure. Uncontrolled diabetes was attributed to nearly half of the newly diagnosed people with CKD. Those with kidney failure required either dialysis or transplantation to live. During 2018, doctors diagnosed almost 132,000 new cases of kidney failure from all causes, although the number of these cases has leveled off relative to the rising population of the United States.

The primary causes of CKD are diabetes, high blood pressure (*hypertension*), glomerular diseases, and cystic diseases, such as polycystic kidney disease (PKD) (chapter 3). The number of people afflicted with these diseases who have progressed to kidney failure are shown in table 1.1. In figure 1.1, you can see the percentage of all people with kidney failure that can be attributed to each cause during the same period. The picture is changing, however, with more new cases being attributed to diabetes (figure 1.2).

Diabetes and hypertension account for 65 percent of the cases of kidney failure. The rest of the cases result from glomerular

TABLE 1.1 Kidney Failure in the United States, 2018

Cause	Number of Cases
Diabetes	304,379
Hypertension	204,889
Glomerular diseases	117,235
Cystic diseases	38,657
All other causes	120,723
Total	785,883

diseases, cystic kidney diseases, and other causes not reflected in figure 1.1 (chapter 3). Alarmingly, the new cases attributed to diabetes and hypertension jumped to 76 percent during 2018 (figure 1.2). Diabetes, the most common cause of kidney failure, accounts for 47 percent of new cases. Because obesity can lead to diabetes and because an increasing number of people are obese or morbidly obese, more people are at risk of CKD and kidney failure. The new cases of kidney failure due to diabetes have accelerated to over sixty-two thousand cases in 2018. Most people are unaware that they even have CKD until later stages of the disease.

Demographically, men have a higher number of total and new cases of kidney failure than women do (figures 1.3 and 1.4),[3] those 45–64 years old and above have a higher number of total and new cases of kidney failure than those under 45 (figures 1.5 and 1.6). Over the past decade, the total number of cases has climbed steadily with a greater increase among the elderly.

Racially, whites have more total cases of kidney failure than do African Americans, Hispanics, and other racial and ethnic groups (figures 1.7 and 1.8). However, these data do not account for the relative size of the population of each group. When this is done, the greatest burden of kidney failure is among Native Hawaiians and Pacific Islanders, being over six times greater than among whites.[4]

FIGURE 1.1. Number of Cases of Kidney Failure in the United States by Disease, 2018

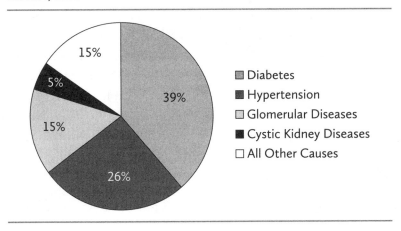

FIGURE 1.2. New Cases of Kidney Failure in the United States by Disease, 2018

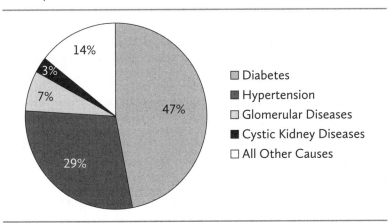

Of the other racial groups, African Americans have the next highest rates, with the rest of the groups having lower rates but all having rates higher than those for whites. Despite this bleak assessment, there is some good news. Native Americans have shown a considerable improvement in the number of total cases over the past decade. In addition, the number of new cases of all minority groups has improved compared to whites. Perhaps, better outreach to these communities has led to better health care among these groups.

Finally, the cost of treating kidney failure has been rising. Much of this cost is born by Medicare. In an era when health care costs are being scrutinized, it is worth mentioning that in 2018 the cost of treating people with CKD and kidney failure in the United States reached more than $131 billion per year in Medicare spending.[3] Those under age 65 can receive Medicare benefits for dialysis and transplantation, adding to the cost. Whether improvements in minority health will ultimately help reduce Medicare expenses, only time will tell.

Disease and Emotions

Discovering that we have a chronic, potentially fatal disease can be overwhelming. It seems that life as we know it has changed, perhaps forever. Sometimes this is true, when we have a disease that doctors can only manage but not treat or cure. Although people with CKD require some form of intervention for their entire lives, doctors can manage *and* treat it.

When I discovered that I had a serious chronic disease, I experienced emotional reactions similar to the six stages of grief related to death as described by Elisabeth Kübler-Ross: fear, denial, anger, bargaining, depression, and, finally, acceptance.[5] Loss of kidney function parallels some aspects of death. CKD can represent the loss of life as we know it. Our reactions might be just as compelling as those people approaching death since we are not sure whether we will survive. My emotional reactions did not necessarily represent a continuum of responses. They came and went over the course of my disease. Even when I finally accepted my disease, occasionally, I became angry and depressed about my condition. At times, I was just tired. However, if I wanted to live, which I did, I *had* to come to terms with all the aspects of CKD.

FIGURE 1.3. Number of Kidney Failure Cases in the United States by Age, 2018

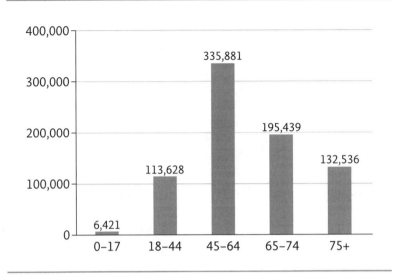

FIGURE 1.4. New Cases of Kidney Failure by Age, 2018

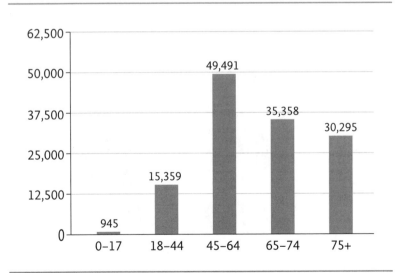

FIGURE 1.5. Number of Kidney Failure Cases in the United States by Gender, 2018

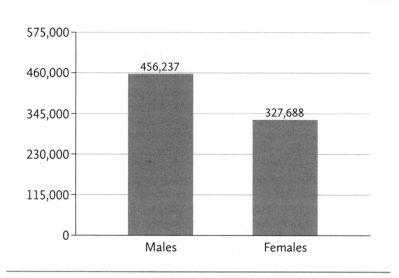

FIGURE 1.6. New Cases of Kidney Failure by Gender, 2018

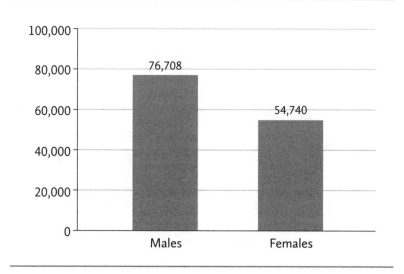

FIGURE 1.7. Number of Kidney Failure Cases in the United States by Race, 2018

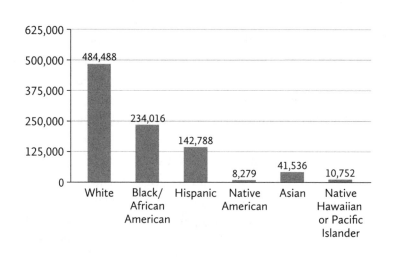

FIGURE 1.8. New Cases of Kidney Failure by Race, 2018

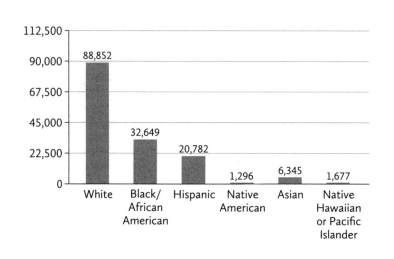

Nearly everyone who has a chronic disease experiences fear and denial. Not knowing what to do can be terrifying and paralyzing. We may know little about our condition and may be afraid of suffering or even dying. Sometimes we may not want to believe that we have a serious illness. People who have spent active lives find it difficult to accept the restrictions placed on activities that are part of life. It is easier to ignore the problem in hopes that the diagnosis is wrong or that the illness will go away.

Yet denial serves a useful purpose by rationing only the amount of information and emotion we can process at any given time. Profound loss is difficult for even the strongest people. Denial gives us time to absorb the news of our illness in a measured way. We cannot believe that our kidneys are failing. We feel fine. Later, the significance of what is happening to us becomes more of a reality.

Once we can no longer deny the fact that we have a chronic illness and the full weight of its reality sinks in, we often become angry. Why me? What did I do to deserve this? Could I have done something to prevent my illness? The questions are endless. You might conclude you have been targeted for illness, possibly as some form of punishment. This is not true. Although contracting an illness is not exactly random—many illnesses are influenced by genetic and lifestyle factors—it is not personal, either. We can imagine all kinds of what-if scenarios. If only we had done something differently, maybe the outcome would have been different. Processing anger can be an important part of emotional healing. Feeling your anger can help you move on.

People who believe in God may try bargaining for a better outcome. If you promise to dedicate the remainder of your life to God's purpose, for example, maybe God will give back your kidney function. In the end, however, it does not matter. The loss is permanent. We must face the reality of our failing kidneys.

When the reality of losing kidney function finally sets in, the emotional responses can deepen, possibly leading to depression, either steady or intermittent. Minor depression—feeling sad—is normal. Like denial, depression can allow the brain time to absorb the full impact of the diagnosis. Eventually, after depression has served its purpose, it can dissipate. But more severe depression can make your treatment more difficult, robbing you of the motivation and energy you need to get treatment and take care of yourself. Depression that does not subside is a very serious condition that may require medical attention. More on depression in chapter 4.

Once you have moved through the stages of fear, denial, anger, bargaining, and depression, you may begin to accept your diagnosis. In time, you will realize that you can no longer avoid kidney disease. It is at this point that you have the greatest opportunity to take control of your health, even if it means your life will never be the same again.

Educating Yourself—and Other Tools for Dealing with Chronic Kidney Disease

Not everyone gets a warning that their kidneys are in danger of failing. Some people discover that they have had high blood pressure for a long time without knowing it. For other people, kidneys fail because of diabetes or other causes that could possibly have been prevented.

In my own case, I lived for twenty years knowing my kidneys might fail, but I seldom thought about it seriously. Because my mother and sister had died of complications of PKD, I knew I might have the disease, but I did not experience symptoms, other than high blood pressure, until I was almost 45 years old. That was the first time I had to confront my own mortality, and it terrified me. Eventually, I had to accept my fate whether I wanted to or not. Acceptance is something that nearly everyone with CKD can achieve.

Like people with other chronic diseases, people with CKD must manage their disease every day for the rest of their lives. There are no days off, and no vacations. If we do not treat our failing kidneys, we can become sicker and possibly die. However, once we learn what to do and integrate those lessons into our lives, our lives can become more normal. Life will not be the same as when we were well, but we can still pursue a happy one. It may not seem that way at this point, but throughout this book, I hope to convince you that your life is not over with CKD, and that other opportunities are possible. I will show you how.

First, learn everything you can about your disease. You may not have a medical background, but you should be able to grasp the basics of your disease when they are described in language you understand. This book will introduce you to information that will allow you to have more control over your condition. I found that the more I understood about CKD, the less afraid I felt.

There are many sources of information about CKD. Start with your doctor. In addition, several kidney disease organizations provide information in accessible language. For more technical information, access the medical literature through the Library of Medicine at the National Institutes of Health in Bethesda, Maryland. (Additional details about such organizations and ways to access the medical literature are provided in the Resources section at the end of this book.)

As I learned more about my disease, I found that I had far less to be concerned about than I thought. There would be tough times, but I knew that with the knowledge that I acquired and with the right attitude, I could make the process of treatment much easier. As a trained scientist, I was able to examine the scientific literature to learn about my disease and I was able to understand what was happening to me. But many scholarly articles are too technical for the nontechnically trained person. One thing I never found was a complete discussion of CKD from a *patient's* point of view. This book aims to fill this void.

I realized early in the progression of my disease that I was ultimately responsible for my health and recovery. I felt that my doctors were my advisors, and that *I* was responsible for following their directions and for the decisions that we ultimately made. If I did not agree with a doctor or was unsure of what to do, I consulted with other doctors until I was convinced that a course of action was right for me. Not everyone has as many options to pursue as I did, but realizing that you always have options to choose from, even if some of them are unattractive, gives you great power.

Before I started dialysis, my doctor had me complete a form outlining several dialysis treatment options. In addition to two types of dialysis, the form gave me the choice of declining dialysis. Declining dialysis would have meant that I would die. Instead, I *chose* to live.

Having choices gives you control. One of the worst aspects of having a chronic disease is feeling helpless and not knowing what to do. Control can seem like merely telling people what to do. However, it is not that simple. Being in control comes from having knowledge of your condition and being able to express your views and pose questions to your doctors and others from a calm, informed perspective. Getting to the point of feeling in control can take time. Keeping an open mind to the possibilities of recovery can help you maintain a positive attitude toward your disease.

Once our kidneys fail, we have only two treatment choices: dialysis (either peritoneal dialysis or hemodialysis) or transplantation. A major issue for people with CKD is deciding which form of treatment is best. Often, we will just accept what our doctors tell us without thinking much about how the treatment will change our lives. I was surprised at how little doctors knew about the day-to-day aspects of living with the treatments they prescribed. For me, it was important to make up my own mind and feel that I had control over what happened to me. I found that feeling in control (or even having the illusion of control) was the most helpful factor in facing CKD. Feeling in control may help you with your chronic illness. Keep in mind that your caregivers also may experience some of the same stresses as you do. Here are some of the lessons I learned.

Coping Skills for Patients and Caregivers

When the reality of CKD set in, I was frightened and didn't know what to do. Over the decade during which my kidneys were progressively failing and at the end of which I received a successful transplant, I learned how to manage my disease. Sometimes it wasn't easy. General information about CKD and treatment options was available, but information about *how* to decide which options to pursue and *how* to adapt to them were not. From my experience, I will share some considerations I had with my disease that I hope will help you with your own experience. First, here are some general coping skills I learned that helped me. They may help you, too.

Move Quickly through Denial and Face Your Disease Directly

I experienced all the emotional reactions to loss, described earlier, to varying degrees, but finally realized that I was ultimately responsible for my health. I had to accept that I was sick. Although the thought was unpleasant and I wanted to hide from it, I was better off confronting my disease. No one would be more motivated than I would be to get well and live as well as I could. In a sense, I felt empowered by accepting my disease. This can be true for you too, although the time needed to reach acceptance may vary.

Be Your Own Advocate

In addition to educating myself about my disease to reduce fear, I found it important to use my knowledge to help my doctors give me the best care possible. Doctors cannot read minds. They often rely on feedback from their patients about how you feel and about reactions to treatments that they prescribe. If you do not tell your doctors about your reactions to their treatments, they will have a more difficult job in treating you. Furthermore, doctors should understand how these treatments affect your life. After all, *you* must live with them. Do not be afraid to ask questions or challenge a treatment option if you think you cannot handle it. If you are too sick to be your own advocate, find someone who can do that for you. It can be a family member or friend. My friends helped me when my condition was very serious.

Doctors do their best to be aware of the latest treatments available for you. However, some new approach may come along that you might want to pursue. Discuss it with your doctor to determine if it might be beneficial for you.

Embrace Your Inner Strength

We each have different personalities and temperaments. On one extreme, some people feel weak and powerless, sensing that they have little control over their lives. Mostly, they depend on others for support and feel that they cannot live without the help of others. At the other extreme, some people feel in total control and independent. They can take on the world and do things with help from relatively few people. Most of us fall between these two extremes.

When adversity strikes, even the strongest of us can question ourselves and doubt our ability to conquer our situation. The weakest can feel even more helpless and hopeless. I was in the middle. I went through many self-doubts when I knew my kidneys would fail. However, I discovered in time that I had a reserve of inner strength that I had not appreciated. To survive psychologically, I had to find that inner strength. I am not sure how I found it, but I think it came from a strong desire to survive. Once I knew I had this inner strength and realized I needed to improve my situation and conquer my disease largely alone, I embraced my strength. You, too, can do it. I have no secret formula, but you will find it, if you allow yourself to look for your inner strength and use it to help you through the difficult times. Some people turn to religion to find the strength, whereas others discover it in their ability to solve their own problems. No matter how you do it, I have learned that finding and embracing your inner strength is worth the journey.

Believe Your Life Will Improve

Having a chronic disease, especially CKD, does not necessarily mean that your life is over. It is amazing how people with the most debilitating diseases or injuries often go on to have fulfilling lives. Take, for example, the late Christopher Reeve, the actor who became quadriplegic after falling from a horse, breaking his neck, and severing his spinal cord. Despite his grave injuries, Reeve passionately believed that he would walk again. He faced his difficult circumstances with courage, dignity, and passion. Although he ultimately died from complications related to his injury, Reeve significantly raised awareness of spinal cord injury and helped increase research funding—accomplishments that must have been very gratifying to him.

What kept me going was the belief that, in the end, I would receive a transplant and my life would be better. I was discouraged from time to time, but I did not lose sight of the goal of receiving a new kidney. I even began planning activities I wanted to pursue, such as traveling the world and even writing books!

Take the Long View

The mind has a way of blurring memories the longer time goes by. My memories of nasty hospital stays or major surgeries faded once I received my kidney transplant. Thus, when I confronted what appeared to be a difficult situation, I looked ahead to the point when my memory would be fuzzy. I believed everything eventually would be okay. When friends of mine face surgery or other traumatic events, I keep reminding them that, in six months, their emotional responses will be considerably less intense than they are at the present.

Remain Optimistic and Give a Positive Spin to Everything

Often there were times when my situation seemed bleak. On a few occasions, there was the possibility that I might not survive. I found it extremely important to believe that I would get better. Although no specific cure was available for PKD, I knew that I could be treated successfully for kidney failure. Whether I remained on dialysis or received a transplant, I believed that I could create a fulfilling life. Regardless of what happened to me, I always tried to look at my situation with optimism. This made my recovery much easier.

Know Your Priorities and Stick to Them

As a kidney dialysis patient, I was continually fatigued, which limited my participation in many activities I enjoyed. Considering the competing demands that I confronted every day, especially at work, I knew that I could not respond to everything. Instead, I developed a list of priorities that were important to me. My health was at the top of the list. Without my health, none of the other priorities mattered. Having priorities helped me decide what I could do or what I could not do. It was very important for me to learn the word *no*. If a request was not consistent with my priorities, I did not feel obliged to accept.

Be Willing to Take Risks

Doctors are not always sure why their patients are sick. They can run a multitude of medical tests, and the cause of the illness still may not be clear. That happened to me when I developed numerous serious infections in 1999. At the time, I was on dialysis. During my many visits to the hospital, my doctors performed all types of procedures to locate the source of infection but to no avail. Many patients with PKD have kidney infections, and medical tests may show some objective diagnostic measures to verify a diagnosis of a kidney infection. For example, blood or urine cultures might have found evidence for bacteria. However, none of my cultures did.

Based on their experience, several nephrologists recommended that I have my kidneys removed. I was not particularly crazy about such a prospect, because I was still passing a fair amount of urine for a person with kidney failure, and having my kidneys removed was life-threatening, major surgery. However, I could not receive a transplant with an active infection, or one suppressed by antibiotics. On the other hand, I could have my kidneys removed and still have the infections. I did not want to place myself at such risk for nothing. It was not a sure thing. But because I wanted a transplant, I felt that I had to take the risk and had both kidneys removed. Fortunately, everything worked out all right. The infections disappeared after the surgeon removed my kidneys, and over the succeeding months, I felt progressively better. The risk ultimately was worth it.

Ask for Help, but Don't Depend on It

When I was very sick, I could not do some things on my own, like driving or shopping. Most of the time, I had friends who could help me when I needed it. However, they were not always available, especially on short notice. I found that it was important to have backup plans, like using taxis or county services for transportation or even a homeworker if needed. Keep in mind that caregivers have lives and responsibilities of their own and may not have endless time and energy to devote to you. I found that if I worked to be independent, even when I felt at my worst, I avoided feeling helpless.

Keep Your Sense of Humor

Someone once said that laughter is the best medicine. I found that to be true as well. Finding the humor in life's challenges can be freeing. For example, many of us in my dialysis center engaged in our own form of humor. In a Frankensteinian sort of way, we would poke fun at all the tubes and gadgets that attached us to dialysis machines. Some people not familiar with dialysis did not understand the humor or were uncomfortable with it. That's okay—even beyond illness, life provides plenty of things to laugh about.

Caregivers

Although we deal with our situations as patients as best we can, often the contributions and sacrifices of caregivers are overlooked and perhaps underappreciated. While I dealt with my CKD, I mostly took care of myself. However, after major surgeries and difficult hospital stays, I had to depend on friends to tend to my needs for a short while. I realized though that I was creating hardships for them. They had their own lives and responsibilities with their own families and careers. In addition, they didn't live nearby. Although I didn't have a constant caregiver, I was aware of the sacrifices they were making and tried to minimize asking them for help.

Many patients with CKD need more care than I did. Some people have live-in families who are available for care. Being on home dialysis requires additional attention by caregivers. In addition, paperwork and phone calls concerning medical insurance can be time consuming and stressful. After consulting several sources, including the National Kidney Foundation and a few of my friends who have been caregivers, I found several valuable coping skills for caregivers.[6]

I thought that caregivers would be constantly under stress but found that they supported their charges out of love. They wanted to do it. But they are human and found themselves periodically feeling overwhelmed.

Many of the coping skills I described for patients also pertain to caregivers. For example, it is useful for caregivers to learn about the disease that their loved ones are experiencing. It helps not only in dealing with doctors but also in helping caregivers empathize with the patient's experiences and feel that they are making a difference.

There are times that patients cannot advocate for themselves. This is an opportunity for caregivers to get the best care for their loved ones. Being educated about CKD helps them be better advocates. From a patient's perspective, it helps to know that the caregiver is sufficiently knowledgeable to take good care of them. That reduces stress on the patient.

Sometimes, it is helpful to know when caregivers are in over their heads and need help. They may need a break and should ask for assistance when they are feeling overwhelmed. In addition, when someone offers to help, let them. Everybody needs a break from a stressful situation to do something just for them. That certainly includes caregivers. In addition, caregivers should take time for themselves and believe that they have a life beyond caregiving. Have a glass of wine or dinner with a friend to recharge and feel that you are in control. Set aside time to be alone and do something enjoyable, such as exercising, reading, meditating, or napping. Get adequate sleep and nutrition. Keep a sense of humor—it benefits the caregiver and the patient. Joke with the patient about everyday problems to relieve tension for everyone.

Finally, connect with other caregivers to deal with their own situation. There is no prior training for caregiving. No one expects to be one. Denial can play a role in being inadequately prepared to be a caregiver. The caregiver role can feel as though it is suddenly thrust on them. As with patients, caregivers can go through the same emotional turmoil of the stages of grief. Again, moving as quickly as possible to acceptance can help in being a better caregiver. Here is where talking to other caregivers can be useful. They can share their experiences and wisdom on how best to approach being a better caregiver. After all, isn't that what they ultimately want for their loved one?

WITH THIS PRELUDE TO CKD, it is almost time to move on to the various aspects of the diseases that can lead to kidney failure. But first, our kidneys are involved in many of the amazing processes that help our bodies function. In the following chapter, we will take a closer look at the kidneys and how they work.

CHAPTER 2

What Kidneys Do

THE KIDNEY IS an exceptionally sophisticated and efficient purification system that cleanses the blood of unwanted by-products produced by the body. (These by-products are called *metabolites*.) Although we have two kidneys, we need only one kidney to live. In fact, people can lose most of their kidney function without becoming ill.

The kidney is bean shaped, approximately the size of an adult's fist, and weighs about half a pound. Located just below the rib cage in the lower back, the two kidneys are not identical. The right one is slightly smaller than the left one to make room for a large lobe of the liver.

Most organs in the body control only one function. The heart pumps blood and the stomach helps digests food. However, kidneys not only filter blood but also regulate several other bodily functions. They

- balance the amount of water and salts (called *electrolytes*) retained by the body,
- control blood pressure,
- maintain the proper balance of acidity in the blood along with the lungs that expel carbon dioxide,
- regulate the production of red blood cells (called *erythrocytes*) that carry oxygen to the various organs of the body,
- control the level of phosphate in the blood, and
- activate vitamin D.

The kidneys function to keep conditions in the body within a normal range, known as *homeostasis*. All of these functions can be affected when kidneys fail.

Filtration

Humans are not the only animals with kidneys. All vertebrates (animals that have a spine) have kidneys. The earliest vertebrates lived in water. Because fish take a lot of water into their bodies, they need a mechanism to eliminate excess amounts. Saltwater fish also require a means to eliminate excess salt that they absorb. If saltwater fish could not expel excess water and salt from their bodies, they would blow up like a balloon and eventually explode. Kidneys may have evolved in animals to regulate water and salt balance.

Kidneys in vertebrates like us also eliminate waste products. Waste products are produced when we digest proteins (such as those found in meat, fish, or dairy products). *Carbohydrates* (sugars and starches) are eventually broken down (metabolized) into water and *carbon dioxide*. However, when glucose (or sugar) exceeds a certain level in the blood, the kidney begins eliminating the excess. When a person's body expels sugar in the urine, it can be a sign that the person has diabetes (see chapter 3).

Kidneys are the body's simple filtration system. A simple system for filtering liquids removes particles greater than a certain size, whether they are coffee grounds or microbes. Filters usually have four parts: (1) a reservoir into which the liquid passes, like a funnel; (2) the filter itself, like porous paper, membranes, or cheesecloth; (3) the funnel stem, like a hose or straw; and (4) a collection receptacle, like a bottle or jar. We use filters every day when we percolate coffee or purify tap water. Most filtration systems use paper or activated charcoal as filters. Kidneys are a bit more complicated, but their filtration system works in a similar way.

Like a simple filtration system, the kidney has four basic parts. Looking at figure 2.1, which compares the kidneys with a funnel, we see that blood containing wastes first enters the kidney from a branch of the renal artery, which is like the reservoir of the funnel. The blood passes through the filtration apparatus, called the *nephron*. Each kidney contains about one million nephrons. Nephrons are composed of the glomerulus, the tubular system, and the collecting duct.

The first part of the nephron is the *glomerulus* (the filter), which has a large surface area to provide efficient filtration. The larger or thicker the filter, the more efficiently it traps bigger particles. The glomerulus allows small molecules to pass through it for further processing while retaining large substances that the body needs, such as various blood cells and protein molecules. In the kidney, filtration occurs as the blood is forced through the walls of the glomerulus and numerous small vessels, through which blood cells cannot pass, into *the tubular system* (the stem of the funnel). Filtration produces a plasma-like fluid called *filtrate*. Substances that the body still needs pass through the glomerulus.

The filtrate leaves the glomerulus and enters the tubules and collecting ducts, where the useful substances are reabsorbed. Unlike the hollow stem of a simple funnel, tubules and collecting ducts are highly complex, with specialized structures that remove waste products while reabsorbing nutrients and salts that the body needs. What is left is urine. The collecting duct connected to the bladder (the collection receptacle, akin to the coffee pot) provides the final filtration step for urine before the body eliminates it.

Let's take a closer look at the tubular system. Tubules attach to the glomerulus and loop through the kidney (figure 2.1). Tubules eliminate *urea*, the main by-product of protein breakdown from the body. However, the body needs some of the salts, water, and other nutrients that also pass from the blood through the glomerulus into the filtrate. The tubules at various points along the loops reabsorb into the capillaries the salts, water, and nutrients the body needs. Excess salts and water not needed by the body remain in the filtrate and are eliminated as urine. So, the entire process of filtration that takes place in the kidneys involves filtering and reabsorbing—until everything useful has been reabsorbed and everything else is sent to the bladder to be eliminated from the body as urine.

FIGURE 2.1. The Filtering Properties of the Kidney

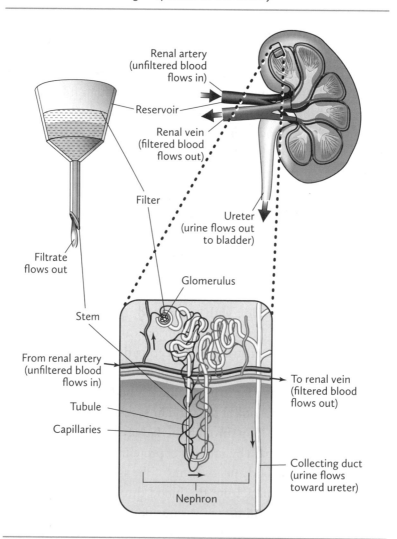

Regulating Blood Pressure

In addition to filtering wastes from blood, kidneys help keep blood pressure from dropping too low. They do this by making and releasing an enzyme called *renin*. Maintaining blood pressure with renin also involves the liver, lungs, and adrenal glands (figure 2.2).

Renin prevents the body from developing dangerously low *sodium* (salt) concentrations. Low sodium leads to low blood pressure. This can occur in hot weather when the body sweats profusely or with substantial blood loss. To prevent low blood pressure during salt depletion, the kidney releases renin into the bloodstream. When renin reaches the liver, it reacts with a protein called *angiotensinogen* to produce a biologically inactive protein called *angiotensin I*.

FIGURE 2.2. How Renin Regulates Blood Pressure

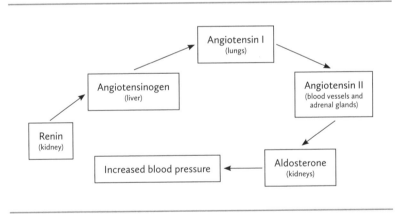

When angiotensin I leaves the liver, it travels to the lungs, where it is converted in the veins to *angiotensin II*. While traveling through the body, angiotensin II constricts blood vessels and raises blood pressure. In addition, angiotensin II acts on the *adrenal glands*, two small endocrine glands, one located on top of each kidney. In the adrenal glands, angiotensin II stimulates the release of the hormone called *aldosterone*, which can direct the kidneys to retain sodium and water. While the right amount of renin at the right time helps maintain blood pressure, it's easy to see how overproduction of renin can contribute to high blood pressure (chapter 3).

Regulating Blood Acidity

The body uses *buffers* to maintain the blood's narrow range of acidity. It is commonly measured as *pH*. pH ranges from 0 to 14, 0 being the most acidic and 14 being the least. A normal pH is 7.0. The buffering process is regulated predominantly by a balance between carbonic acid and bicarbonate (baking soda) in the blood and by the acidity of the urine. In the kidney, carbonic acid flowing along the tubular membrane swaps places with sodium (one of the salts) and bicarbonate. The lungs help to balance bicarbonate levels by releasing carbon dioxide. Various conditions can change the acidity of the blood. If you breathe hard and fast, the blood can become less acidic because of a reduction of carbon dioxide. If the kidney does not function properly, acid can accumulate, a condition known as *acidosis*.

Producing Red Blood Cells

Bone marrow makes red blood cells, which carry oxygen throughout the body. Red blood cells live about four months and then must be replaced. The kidneys produce a hormone called *erythropoietin*, which controls the rate at which red blood cells form. When the kidney senses too little oxygen in the blood, it releases erythropoietin to stimulate the bone marrow to make more red blood cells. When kidney function is degraded or lost and the kidneys make insufficient erythropoietin, patients may have too few red blood cells, a condition called *anemia*.

Regulating Phosphate

Phosphate is essential for the body to produce energy. Dairy products are a major source of phosphate. Numerous chemical reactions in the body use phosphate, but our diets generally provide more phosphate than we need. The kidney is the only means of eliminating excess phosphate carried in the blood. If the kidney malfunctions, several problems can result from an excess of phosphate.

For example, phosphate readily combines with *calcium*. When excess phosphate binds to enough calcium, the body thinks it does not have enough calcium in the blood, prompting bones to release calcium into the bloodstream. When calcium is released into the bloodstream, people may develop *bone disorders* and form calcium phosphate plaques in their organs, possibly leading to organ failure (see chapter 4).

Regulating Bone Structure

Excess phosphate in the blood is not the only cause of bone demineralization. *Vitamin D,* a fat-soluble vitamin, plays an important role in the body's absorption of calcium to maintain strong bones and teeth. Making vitamin D is a complicated process involving active and less active forms of vitamin D (figure 2.3).

FIGURE 2.3. How Vitamin D Is Produced

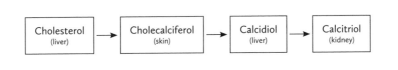

The body makes active forms of vitamin D from *cholesterol*. One mechanism requires sunlight, which stimulates the formation of *cholecalciferol*, a derivative of cholesterol, in the skin. Activated cholecalciferol then passes through the liver and becomes an even more active form of vitamin D called *calcidiol*. The final activation of vitamin D occurs in the kidney. When calcidiol enters the kidney, it is converted to *calcitriol*, the only form of vitamin D that the body actually uses. Some dietary supplements contain cholecalciferol, bypassing the need for the sun's activation of less active forms of vitamin D. Failing kidneys may affect the body's ability to absorb vitamin D, which can lead to bone loss.

MANY OF THE BODY'S essential activities depend on normal kidney function. When kidneys fail, there are major consequences for the body. In the following chapter, we discuss why kidneys may fail.

CHAPTER 3

Why Kidneys Fail

NUMEROUS HEALTH PROBLEMS can lead to chronic kidney disease (CKD). The four main causes are diabetes, hypertension, glomerular diseases, and polycystic kidney disease (PKD). Genetics plays a role in most causes of CKD and is the primary cause of PKD. Genetics is not the whole story, however. Lifestyle and other environmental factors may also be significant contributors. This chapter begins with a primer on the genetic and environmental factors contributing to CKD. Knowledge of these factors will help you understand how you might slow the progression of your disease.

Nature versus Nurture

Genetic Factors

All the functions in our bodies operate based on instructions embedded in our genetic code. Over the past seventy years, researchers have uncovered the intricate details of how this genetic code works. The Human Genome Project, which was completed in 2003, determined the complete nucleotide sequence of human *deoxyribonucleic acid (DNA)*.

Genes provide a blueprint for creating our bodies and making them work. Just as the blueprints for a house show how to build its various parts, such as the foundation, walls, and roof, genes direct the construction of cells, organs, bone, and skin. Moreover, like the heating, air-conditioning, and electrical systems that control the environmental conditions in a house, genes control how our bodies function.

The primary purpose of genes is to make *proteins*. Proteins are like a building's construction workers and engineers. They make and operate the human body according to the genetic blueprints residing within the *chromosomes*.

While we are in the womb, our genes issue the instructions (or blueprints) to make proteins, which leads to the formation of all the organs of the body. For organs to develop correctly, certain processes must happen in an exact way. It starts when a sperm fertilizes the egg. The cells in the resulting embryo, possessing two copies of each gene, one from each parent, begin to divide. As the embryo grows, copies of genes inherited from each parent must be reproduced identically in each new cell, so that all the cells in the developing fetus (and eventually in the person's body) will have the same set of genetic blueprints.

Although rare, mistakes can occur when genes are copied. Called *mutations*, these mistakes can cause the organs to work improperly. If a house's blueprints are wrong, a door might be in the wrong place or the lighting system might fail because of incorrect wiring. In people, when genetic mistakes in the egg and sperm of parents are passed along to their children, they can cause them to inherit a disease. For example, mutations in genes that make or control kidneys can cause the genes to malfunction, leading to kidney disease.

Environmental Factors

Behavioral and environmental factors can also contribute to the expression or progression of a disease. In the case of CKD, an improper diet, lack of exercise, and other lifestyle factors can contribute greatly to a person's medical status. We do not deliberately set out to make ourselves ill. However, with the stresses of our culture and of everyday life, it can be easy to neglect our own health.

Between work, family, and social obligations, we are so busy that we may have little time to eat properly or to get adequate exercise. Over time, our health can begin to fail without our even knowing it.

When people don't eat right and don't exercise, they are more likely to be overweight or obese. Obesity has reached epidemic proportions in the United States and in other countries.[1] According to the World Health Organization, the rates of overweight or obesity have almost tripled worldwide since 1975 to 48 percent in 2016. In the United States, the rates are similar.[2] Obesity may lead to other health complications—including CKD—because obesity makes people more likely to develop diabetes and hypertension. Excess weight can also cause coronary heart disease, high cholesterol levels, and stroke, which can lead to death.

Diseases That Cause Kidney Failure

References to the symptoms of kidney disorders by the ancient Greeks suggest that we have known about CKD for thousands of years. We couldn't analyze kidneys and other organs until the nineteenth century, however. In 1827, the English physician Richard Bright first described the symptoms of CKD.

In the twenty-first century, CKD is still incurable, but it can be prevented and treated. With dialysis and transplantation, people with CKD can continue to have productive lives. Nevertheless, failing kidneys take a very high medical, emotional, and financial toll. Even though there is no cure for CKD, knowing its causes can help you prevent, delay, or prepare for it.

As we learned in chapter 1, over 786,000 people in the United States are living with CKD. In most cases, diabetes and hypertension are the causes, and both are preventable (chapter 5). Glomerular disorders, which can have both environmental and genetic origins, are another cause of CKD. There are also inherited causes of CKD, such as PKD. If a person inherits certain mutated genes,

PKD will develop, although the progression of the disease varies among families and individuals. This chapter presents a brief overview of each of these four leading causes of CKD and a few other lesser known ones.

Diabetes

Diabetes (also known as diabetes mellitus) is the leading cause of CKD globally. According to the WHO, the number of people having diabetes increased almost fourfold from 1980 to 2014, affecting 8.5 percent of the world's population.[3] Although most people with diabetes are adults, the disease is rising among children. Worldwide, diabetes is the leading cause of CKD. In the United States, diabetes accounts for 39 percent of cases of kidney failure (figure 1.1). Because of rising obesity rates, the total number of cases of diabetes is increasing as well, even among obese children. Over thirty-four million people over the age of 18 had diabetes in 2018.[4] As people age, they become more susceptible to diabetes (figure 3.1), and almost 27 percent of all people with diabetes are 65 years or older. However, new cases reflect a different pattern. Those 45 to 64 years old have the highest number of cases, which may reflect that younger people are living longer to older ages. Those with less than a high school diploma and/or who are living in low- to middle-income countries also have a higher prevalence of diabetes. Across the American population, slightly more men than women have diabetes. Racially, diabetes affects disproportionately Native Americans, non-Hispanic African Americans, and Hispanic Americans (figure 3.2). Asians on the average have a slightly increased risk for diabetes, compared to non-Hispanic whites. However, the number of new cases is highest in Asian Indians among the Asian American population. New cases are highest among Hispanics and non-Hispanic African Americans, compared to non-Hispanic whites. With the high prevalence of diabetes globally, understanding the underlying causes of diabetes is essential for learning how to prevent and treat it.

FIGURE 3.1. Estimated Number of Cases of Diabetes in People Aged 18 Years and Older, by Age Group, United States, 2020

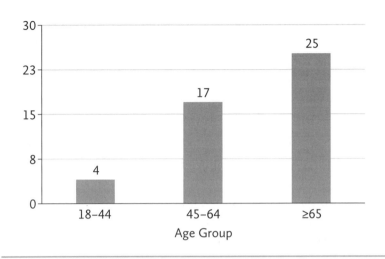

Source: National Diabetes Statistics Report, 2020 estimates of total prevalence (both diagnosed and undiagnosed were projected to year 2018).

FIGURE 3.2. Estimated Age-Adjusted Number of Cases of Diabetes in People Aged 18 Years and Older, by Race/Ethnicity, United States, 2020

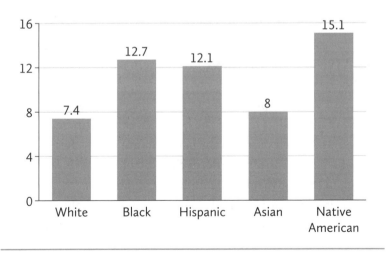

Source: National Diabetes Statistics Report, 2020 estimates of total prevalence (both diagnosed and undiagnosed were projected to year 2018). White, Black, and Asians are non-Hispanic. Native Americans include American Indians and Alaskan Natives.

Diabetes is a metabolic disease in which the body does not properly use glucose. *Glucose* is the main source of energy in the body. For glucose to enter cells, the pancreas secretes the protein *insulin* from beta cells into the bloodstream. The circulating insulin helps glucose cross the membranes surrounding cells. If this process is interrupted, glucose accumulates in the blood and can spill out into the urine. Cells can starve without glucose, even with high concentrations of glucose in the blood, if the glucose cannot cross the cell membranes. The inability of insulin to facilitate glucose transport into cells can occur for one of two reasons: (1) not enough insulin secretion by the pancreas or (2) cells don't respond to insulin, which is called *insulin resistance*.

Type 1 Diabetes. When the pancreas does not secrete enough insulin, this condition is known as type 1 diabetes, sometimes called juvenile diabetes, because it is generally seen in children. Attacks from the body's own immune system destroy beta cells, thereby reducing insulin secretion. Globally, 10–15 percent of people with diabetes have type 1. It is highest in the Scandinavian countries followed by the United Kingdom, North America, and Australia.[5] Type 1 diabetes is lowest in China, Korea, and Japan. These differences are largely because of variations in genetic makeup between these two populations. In the United States, 5 percent of people with diabetes have type 1 diabetes, which usually develops in childhood.[4] Type 1 diabetes is more prevalent in whites than in people of other races.

Type 1 diabetes progresses in three stages.[6] It begins with the release of antibodies against the beta cells of the pancreas. As the antibodies do their damage, the beta cells are slowly destroyed. Finally, the lack of insulin results in elevated blood levels of glucose, leading to hyperglycemia, the hallmark of diabetes.

Researchers have found that type 1 diabetes develops because of genetic and environmental factors. Up to 50 percent of people with type 1 diabetes have the disease because of genetic susceptibility—they inherited an increased likelihood of developing it.

Many genetic risk factors involving the immune system are needed for type 1 diabetes to develop. However, the genetic factors alone are not enough. Scientists believe that environmental triggers, such as prenatal events, viral infections, diet, environmental toxins, psychological stress, and even the season of the year can precipitate type 1 diabetes. Perhaps, the overuse of antibiotics altering the microbial environment in the gut and the immune system may trigger type 1 diabetes.[7] A more complete and detailed discussion can be found elsewhere.[8]

People with type 1 diabetes must take insulin to live. Although several methods for administering insulin have become available (chapter 5), the cost of insulin has skyrocketed, doubling from 2012 to 2016.[9] This problem has put people's lives at risk, when the cost of insulin begins competing with other necessities of life, such as rent and food. Over the past couple of years, price increases have steadied because of pressure from the federal government. How the problem will resolve itself remains to be seen.

Type 2 Diabetes. The number one cause of CKD is type 2 diabetes. Type 2 diabetes accounts for most cases of diabetes and is clearly linked to obesity. Almost 80 percent of people with type 2 diabetes are overweight.[2] In type 2 diabetes, although the pancreas secretes plenty of insulin, the cells of the body become resistant to it, preventing the transport of glucose into the cells. Like people with type 1 diabetes, people with type 2 diabetes also may need insulin supplementation to live. Mild cases of type 2 diabetes, however, can usually be controlled through diet and oral, noninsulin medications.

Type 2 diabetes is much more prevalent in minority populations, largely because these groups have higher rates of obesity. Native Americans have one of the highest rates of type 2 diabetes in the world. Other minority groups greatly affected by type 2 diabetes include African Americans, non-Hispanic African Americans, and Hispanic Americans. Because of the high rates of obesity in these populations, the US Centers for Disease Control and Prevention expects the rates of diabetes to increase in the future. Indeed, children and young adults are showing increased rates of type 2 diabetes, now surpassing their rates of type 1 diabetes.[10] A recent study indicates that those who develop type 2 diabetes at a young age are at higher risk for kidney failure than those who develop the disease at an older age.[11]

Diabetes can create many complications affecting almost every part of the body. In addition to CKD, diabetes can lead or contribute to heart and blood vessel disease, strokes, blindness, limb amputations, nerve damage, and brain disorders, including cognitive decline, dementia, even Alzheimer's disease, especially in the elderly. Moreover, babies born to women with uncontrolled diabetes can have birth defects. This is all a big price to pay for a disease that is preventable in most cases by maintaining a normal weight. Medical researchers are working hard to identify the hormonal and environmental causes of increasing rates of obesity and to develop treatments and programs to conquer the obesity epidemic. (See discussions that follow about hormones and obesity and obesity and diabetes.)

Type 2 diabetes has a poorly understood genetic component. Research is under way to determine which genes are involved and to what extent they play a role in the development of the disease. Having answers to these questions will help doctors identify who is most susceptible to diabetes and locate potential targets for treatment.

Type 2 diabetes can run in families. However, the genetic basis of the mutations that lead to diabetes varies among family members. Thus, numerous genes may be responsible for an increased susceptibility to type 2 diabetes. Although researchers have studied so-called *polygenetic diseases* for more than thirty years, they have learned that finding the genes that contribute the most to a disease is quite difficult. Type 2 diabetes is no exception, especially considering the importance of environment and lifestyle in the disease. This does not mean that scientific research has yielded no new information about the genetic contribution to diabetes. Quite the contrary! Researchers have made a good start in identifying the genes involved.

Many international genetic studies have examined the genes involved in insulin secretion from pancreatic cells as well as how insulin acts on cells in the body.[12] These studies found more than eighty genetic variants in diabetic populations, most of which regulate insulin secretion and a few that regulate insulin sensitivity. Each one of these variants contributes only small amounts to the predisposition for the disease. It is not known whether any of these variants will lead to a better understanding of the disease or to a novel approach for treating type 2 diabetes. More extensive research is required.

Understanding the relationship between obesity and type 2 diabetes is critical. In the United States, 78 percent of Americans are overweight, obese, or morbidly obese;[2] African Americans and Hispanic Americans have a higher prevalence of obesity than non-Hispanic whites. Moreover, women across all races are more obese than men. Obesity increases with age, leveling off by age 60 or declining thereafter. With the increase in obesity and type 2 diabetes in children, it is important to understand the possible relationships between these two diseases to avoid surges in diabetes later in life.[13] The key to these relationships may be in the way the brain interacts and modifies the body's response to too much glucose. Here's how.

Researchers have learned a great deal about the variety of substances that control appetite, including hormones.[14] *Hormones* act on receptors to exert their functions. One of these functions is appetite. *Receptors* are specialized entities on surfaces of cell membranes that react specifically to only one hormone, similarly structured hormones, or synthetic compounds. Think of the hormone-receptor interaction as a key and a lock. Only one key (or keys very similar to it) will unlock the door so the hormone will respond appropriately.

One such hormone, called *leptin*, regulates appetite through an interaction with a receptor. When blood leptin levels are high, we eat less, and when they are low, we eat more. Normally, when we eat, leptin levels increase, telling us that we're full. However, if leptin receptors do not respond appropriately, we can eat more food despite being full, and obesity can result. Obese people often have higher leptin levels, which correlate with insulin resistance. If leptin receptors respond less to a given amount of leptin, the body then secretes more of it.

Another factor in insulin resistance resides in the brain, specifically in an area called the *hypothalamus*.[14] This brain area regulates food intake by responding to levels of insulin and leptin in the blood, as well as to glucose and certain types of fat called free fatty acids. When the brain detects that the actions of these hormones are sufficient, it tells us to eat less food. Conversely, when these signals are in short supply, the brain tells us to eat more food. Recent research implicates other areas of the brain in this process that may play a role in our feeling hungry and in deciding to eat.[15] So, if brain mechanisms can no longer keep food intake within normal limits, weight gain and insulin resistance can result. How does this happen?

It turns out that the brain has insulin receptors that can become resistant to insulin, just as those in peripheral tissues can. In fact, the biochemical pathways that mediate the actions of insulin appear to be similar in both the brain and peripheral tissues. Like peripheral tissues, the brain receptors become more resistant to insulin with excess food intake. Thus, the brain's control of food intake is impaired, resulting in obesity. The brain responds to leptin in the same way as tissues do elsewhere in the body. Thus, obesity can lead to type 2 diabetes by a multifaceted process.

To sum up, when we eat, food is partially converted into glucose to feed the body's cells and to provide the energy they need to operate. To transport glucose into the cells, the pancreas secretes insulin, thereby regulating our blood levels of glucose. If we eat too much food over a long period, the cells, including those in the brain, become resistant to the constant bombardment of too much insulin. In addition, the release of leptin to control our food intake no longer controls our appetite, and we develop resistance to leptin. Finally, when insulin production is insufficient to move glucose into cells, glucose rises to dangerous levels in the blood and can result in type 2 diabetes.

We have seen that many altered physiological mechanisms can lead to obesity and diabetes. Genetic variants, too, might contribute to the ultimate expression of type 2 diabetes.[16] Several variants for obesity have been identified, but their exact role in its development is not yet known. A genetic role for retaining fat could make sense from an evolutionary perspective. When food was scarce in ancient times, there could be a survival advantage for those who retained fat.[17] They would have more energy stores than those without such genetic variants to withstand long periods without food. Now, the plentiful supply of food in developed countries would render such genetic variants for retaining fat a disadvantage. Once the genetic role of obesity is better characterized, researchers can compare variants with those for type 2 diabetes, which may help clarify the role of obesity in type 2 diabetes.

One last point about obesity and type 2 diabetes. Up to 30 percent of obese people are metabolically healthy with normal insulin sensitivity. It is easy to think that someone in that category is not at risk of developing type 2 diabetes. However, research has found that this group has a significantly elevated chance of developing diabetes.[18] Thus, it is important that obese, metabolically healthy people be followed by their health care team for signs of diabetes and to encourage weight loss.

Finally, two other factors may contribute to type 2 diabetes: inflammation and intestinal bacteria. Accumulating evidence suggests that inflammation may ultimately contribute to developing type 2 diabetes[19] and may result from a high-fat diet.[20] Inflammation can be good when fighting infections but not so good when done to excess. These results suggest that those with type 2 diabetes should reduce the amount of fat in their diets to keep inflammation in check.

Our intestines contain a host of bacteria called the *microbiome*. The composition of these bacteria is altered in those with type 2 diabetes.[21] Emerging research has suggested that improving the bacterial environment to a healthier one might help reverse the consequences of type 2 diabetes. Indeed, using bariatric surgery to reverse the disease (chapter 5) appears to shift the bacterial environment from an unhealthy to a healthy intestinal composition.[22] Thus, using such approaches, such as eating yogurt or taking probiotics, might be helpful. Check with your doctor to determine if this approach might be useful to you.

How does diabetes lead to CKD? The process, technically known as *diabetic nephropathy*, typically develops over a period of ten to twenty-five years. It starts when excess glucose in the blood degrades the filtering capacity of the glomerulus in the kidney (chapter 2). Normally, the glomerulus will allow only small molecules, such as water and salts, to pass through, leaving behind large molecules like proteins. When protein is excreted in the urine, a condition called *albuminuria* is often the first sign of diabetes. (A *sign* is something a doctor can identify through testing. A *symptom* is something the patient experiences or notices.) Kidney function is generally normal at this stage. However, if the deterioration of the filtration of blood through the glomerulus continues, increasing amounts of protein pass into the urine and cause scarring of the glomerulus, leading to declining kidney function.

How high glucose concentrations degrade kidney function is not completely understood. Aggravating factors that can accelerate the decline of kidney function are high blood pressure, high cholesterol, obesity, and smoking.[23] Even high blood glucose levels in prediabetes may begin damaging kidneys.[24] Fortunately, these are factors that can be reduced with appropriate treatment. In addition, researchers have discovered a number of potential biochemical pathways that are stimulated by glucose, such as inflammatory pathways. These pathways seem to underlie the growth of some cells in the glomerulus and tubules that lead to scarring and fiber-like tissue, thereby degrading kidney function. If these processes continue long enough, CKD and kidney failure can result.

Hypertension

Hypertension, or high blood pressure, is the second leading cause of CKD, accounting for 26 percent of cases in the United States. Blood pressure that is too high can damage kidneys and cause them to ultimately fail. (High blood pressure is defined below.)

Like diabetes, hypertension is a worldwide problem. According to the American Heart Association Statistical 2018 Update,[25] global prevalence of hypertension increased from 605 million to 978 million from 1980 to 2008 and was a major cause of premature death by 2015, according to the WHO. By 2010, it was the leading risk factor for heart disease and stroke. Africa (especially South Africa),[26] along with Eastern Europe and Central Asia, had the highest rates of hypertension, which were greatest in low- to middle-income countries. In such countries, treatment is either not available, not affordable, or both, explaining why hypertension rates are so high.[27]

In the United States, 34 percent of adults have hypertension (figure 1.1), with men and women having similar rates. The percentage of the population having high blood pressure increases with age, the highest rates being in those 75 and older. African Americans have the highest rates of hypertension, and it has been increasing in that demographic from 1988 through 2014.[25] To prevent the medical consequences of high blood pressure, including CKD, effective treatment of it is paramount.

To understand high blood pressure, it is necessary to first understand what blood pressure is and what values are considered high. When the heart pumps blood through the blood vessels, the blood pushing against the walls of these vessels increases the pressure. Two numbers express this pressure: one is pressure when the heart has contracted (known as maximum, or *systolic*, pressure), and the other is the pressure after the heart relaxes (known as minimum, or *diastolic*, pressure).

Blood pressure can be measured using a blood pressure monitor. A blood pressure cuff is wrapped around the upper arm. The cuff is inflated using a pump until the pulse in the upper arm is no longer heard. The cuff is slowly deflated until the sounds of heartbeats return. The pressure at which the sounds are first heard is the systolic pressure, whereas the pressure at which sounds are no longer detectable is the diastolic pressure. The blood pressure monitor provides a readout of two numbers. The measured blood pressure is expressed as a ratio of these two numbers, like 120/80 (systolic/diastolic, or "systolic over diastolic").

Care must be taken to get an accurate blood pressure reading. To that end, the American Heart Association recommends several steps that should be taken:

1. Remain still for the time necessary for blood pressure to be at a normal, nonactive level. Often in a doctor's office, a nurse will immediately take your body pressure as soon as you sit down. This is not enough time for the body to be in a resting state.
2. Be sure to sit correctly with both feet flat on the floor on a hard chair with your arm with the cuff on a flat surface. This is especially important when taking blood pressures at home.
3. Take blood pressure measurements at the same time of day. They can vary throughout the day.
4. Take multiple readings and record the results.
5. Make sure that no clothing is between the skin and the cuff.

Blood pressures are usually taken with an automatic blood pressure monitor. It pumps up the cuff until the detector cannot "hear" the heartbeat and then releases the pressure cuff until the heartbeat can no longer be heard. A word of caution: some people find that the automatic machines measure the systolic pressure as higher than what would be found after a manual check. If an automatic machine measures your systolic pressure as above normal, have it checked again manually to make sure the measurement is accurate.

A blood pressure at or below 120/80 is considered normal. Higher values may be evidence of high blood pressure, or *hypertension*. Hypertension is categorized as more or less severe based on the degree of pressure elevation. Recently, the criteria for determining high blood pressure has been controversial. According to the National Institutes of Health (NIH), if the systolic pressure reaches 120 to 139 or the diastolic pressure reaches 80 to 89, a person is prehypertensive. People with systolic pressures of 140 and above, or diastolic pressures of 90 or above, are considered hypertensive. In either case, medications and/or lifestyle changes are necessary to control blood pressure. However, a consortium of the American College of Cardiology, the American Heart Association, and others recommends lower values: <120/<80 is considered normal, 120–129/<80 is elevated, 130–139/80–89 is stage 1 hypertensive, and ≥140/≥90 is stage 2 hypertensive.[28] In the two hypertensive stages, if either the systolic or diastolic pressure meet the criterion, a person is considered hypertensive. Other groups have created their own guidelines that will not be discussed here.

The NIH's and cardiologists' criteria on the percentage of people who are hypertensive are compared in figures 3.3–3.6. Not surprisingly, in all cases, the percentage of those meeting the lower hypertension criterion (from the cardiologists) is greater than those meeting the higher one (from the NIH). This can be seen for both men and women, as well as when comparing different races or ethnicities. Note that up to age 65, a higher percentage of men are hypertensive compared to women, and then women catch up to men and exceed them by age 75. Consistent with these results, recent research indicates that women begin having high blood pressure earlier than men and a steeper increase over time that continues throughout life.[29] African American men and women have a higher prevalence of high blood pressure than Asians, Hispanics, and non-Hispanic whites. One reason that African Americans have a higher risk for hypertension may be genetic differences that will be discussed later in this chapter. So, which of the criteria should you choose? The answer depends on the form of kidney disease you have and, therefore, the best choice for blood pressure control is best left to a discussion with your health care team. This is particularly true in the elderly, who may be too frail for aggressive blood pressure control.

Two factors contribute to the development of hypertension: (1) the amount of blood flowing through a vessel and (2) the vessel's diameter (figure 3.7). These factors affect either the systolic or the diastolic pressure. The amount of blood flowing through blood vessels results from the volume of blood leaving the heart with each contraction and the heart rate. The higher the volume of blood expelled or the higher the heart rate, the higher the systolic blood pressure. The diameter of the blood vessels affects blood pressure by resisting blood flow. The smaller the diameter of the vessels, the higher the diastolic blood pressure. This is analogous to running water though a hose and putting your thumb over the nozzle. Constricting the hose nozzle with your thumb, you can feel the water pressure build. One reason that vessels may be small is because of blockages due to *atherosclerosis* (a buildup of plaque within the vessels). There are other reasons, such as eating too much salt, advancing age, and obesity. The particular cause of hypertension determines the appropriate medical treatment (chapter 5).

Physiological factors such as varying heart rate and the muscular tone of blood vessels aren't the only things that influence blood pressure. Genetic susceptibility may also influence a person's blood pressure. Just as in diabetes research, determining which specific genes are responsible for blood pressure and their relative contribution to hypertension has been difficult. As we learned in chapter 2, the renin-angiotensin system is a hormonal system that regulates blood pressure. It evolved to combat dehydration by

FIGURE 3.3. Number of Cases of Hypertension by Age for Men Using ≥130/80 and ≥140/90 as Blood Pressure Standards, United States, 2014

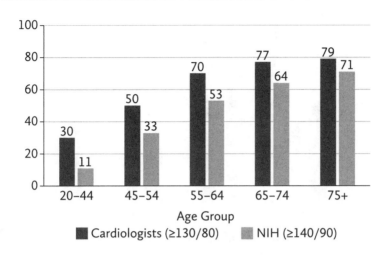

Source: 2017 ACC/AHA/AAPA/ABC/ACPM/AGS/APhA/ASH/ASPC/NMA/PCNA guideline for the prevention, detection, evaluation, and management of high blood pressure in adults.

FIGURE 3.4. Number of Cases of Hypertension by Age for Women Using ≥130/80 and ≥140/90 as Blood Pressure Standards, United States, 2014

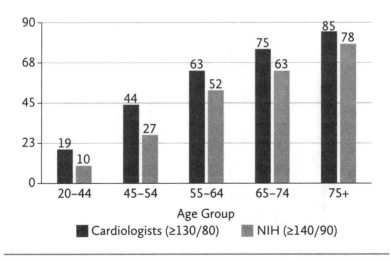

Source: 2017 ACC/AHA/AAPA/ABC/ACPM/AGS/APhA/ASH/ASPC/NMA/PCNA guideline for the prevention, detection, evaluation, and management of high blood pressure in adults.

FIGURE 3.5. Number of Cases of Hypertension by Race/Ethnicity for Men Using ≥130/80 and ≥140/90 as Blood Pressure Standards, United States, 2014

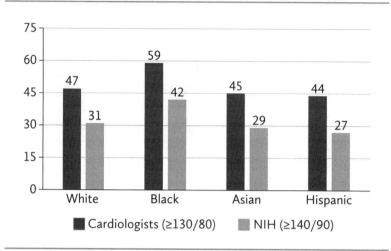

Source: 2017 ACC/AHA/AAPA/ABC/ACPM/AGS/APhA/ASH/ASPC/NMA/PCNA guideline for the prevention, detection, evaluation, and management of high blood pressure in adults. White, black, and Asians are non-Hispanic.

FIGURE 3.6. Number of Cases of Hypertension by Race/Ethnicity for Women Using ≥130/80 and ≥140/90 as Blood Pressure Standards, United States, 2014

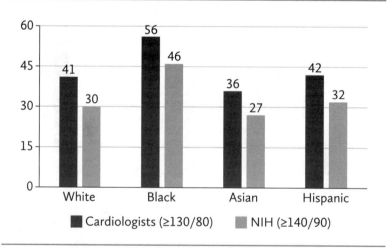

Source: 2017 ACC/AHA/AAPA/ABC/ACPM/AGS/APhA/ASH/ASPC/NMA/PCNA guideline for the prevention, detection, evaluation, and management of high blood pressure in adults. White, black, and Asians are non-Hispanic.

FIGURE 3.7. Factors in High Blood Pressure

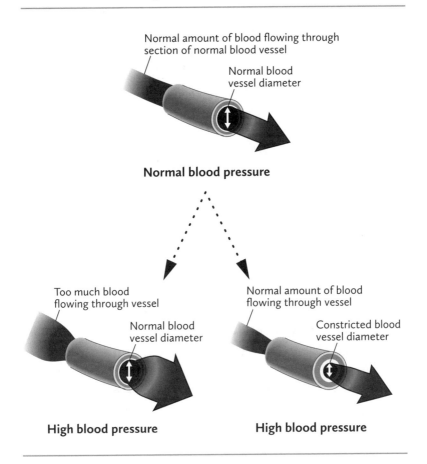

retaining sodium and maintaining blood pressure when the body loses sodium. In this system alone, it is possible that many genes could be altered in a way that promotes hypertension. Indeed, genetic researchers have identified over five hundred candidate genes, with twenty-one looking the most promising.[30] These candidate genes are involved with the renin-angiotensin system and salt sensitivity.

As already discussed, eating too much salt can lead to hypertension. However, each person responds to salt differently. Some people are very sensitive to salt, whereas some are insensitive. These differences suggest that salt sensitivity has a genetic component. A high sensitivity to salt to increase blood pressure is an advantage in hot, dry climates, where it is easy to become dehydrated. Sensitivity to salt is especially a problem for African Americans, which contributes to their hypertension. It accounts for much of the racial differences between African Americans and whites.[31] One genetic difference appears to involve channels through which sodium is reabsorbed in the kidneys, with enhanced sodium and water retention as a result.[32] Another genetic difference may involve hormones called *natriuretic peptides*. These hormones play a role in salt-sensitive hypertension. African Americans have significantly lower blood concentrations of these peptides than whites do.[33] This finding may also explain why high blood pressure is so high in Africa.

At this point, with so many genes possibly involved, researchers do not expect that a mutation in a single gene will be responsible for hypertension. More likely, the interplay of many genes promotes hypertension. Environment and lifestyle can also contribute to hypertension through a complex gene-environment interaction. One example of this type of interaction is excessive salt (sodium) intake and retention, especially for African Americans. Risk factors include aging, family history, gender, and unhealthy lifestyles, such as obesity and smoking.

Research on genes underlying hypertension is still in its infancy and will require many more studies to identify the specific genes responsible. Future research may also yield new medications to reduce hypertension. Because hypertension plays such an important role in kidney disease, these new medications may give physicians better tools to prevent or reduce the progression of CKD.

Obesity and Hypertension. Obesity contributes to hypertension as well as diabetes. Recently, the problem of obesity has extended to children who are now at risk for hypertension and CKD, making the search for ways to reduce obesity more acute.[34]

Obese people often take in an excessive amount of salt, which can lead to hypertension. The high pressure on the glomerulus can slowly degrade its filtering capacity and precipitate reactions such as those that occur in diabetes-induced CKD. In addition, accumulating fat, especially abdominal (belly) fat, can contribute to hypertension. Considering that obesity, hypertension, and diabetes often accompany one another, it can be hard to know which problem came first. However, obesity is often the primary cause of hypertension and diabetes.

Accumulating evidence suggests that the brain plays a role in high blood pressure in obese people.[35] Leptin, the hormone that regulates hunger and may be involved in the development of diabetes, as discussed earlier in this chapter, elevates blood pressure by acting on the hypothalamus. But since leptin acts through several different biochemical pathways, it isn't known whether hypertension and diabetes develop because of changes to the same leptin-involved mechanisms. More research is needed to clarify this issue.

Other brain mechanisms may also be involved in hypertension. For example, *vasopressin*, a hormone that regulates salt and water balance, may be unable to keep up with a constant bombardment of salt.[36] Normally, vasopressin is released when salt concentrations rise to both retain water and to prevent hypertension. However, over time, its actions can be reduced allowing blood pressure to increase. Another mechanism is the renin-angiotensin system that stimulates nerves in the brain to control blood pressure.[37] Normally, this system works to maintain a normal blood pressure. However, when it is overactive, hypertension results. With more research, these mechanisms may suggest potential therapeutic possibilities.

We know that hypertension slowly destroys the kidneys' ability to filter the blood, but how does hypertension lead to kidney failure? With prolonged hypertension, the excess pressure can injure small blood vessels in the kidney and can destroy the filtering ability of the glomerulus (chapter 2), leading to CKD. Using the hose metaphor, if you attach cheesecloth tightly over the end of the hose, water will flow through the cheesecloth without harming it. But if you pinch the hose, increasing the flow pressure, the cheesecloth will begin to degrade and eventually rupture.

Glomerular Diseases

Glomerular diseases are a complex set of disorders. The three main causes of glomerular diseases are autoimmune diseases, hereditary nephritis, and infections. They are the third leading cause of CKD in the United States, accounting for 15 percent of cases (figure 1.1). They are also a worldwide problem.[38] Of the diseases discussed in this section, focal segmental glomerulosclerosis (FSGS) is most prevalent in the United States and Canada, lupus nephritis and FSGS in Latin America, IgA nephropathy and FSGS in Europe, and lupus nephritis in Asia. Glomerular diseases often result in inflammation of the glomerulus, which can eventually cause the formation of scar tissue. As a result, protein leaks into the urine instead of being absorbed back into the blood circulation. Sometimes, glomerular diseases are collectively referred to as *nephrotic syndrome*, because the diseases attack and scar the glomerulus. Like diabetes and hypertension, glomerular diseases slowly destroy the filtering ability of the glomerulus. Excess pressure on the sensitive glomerulus can lead to CKD.

Focal Segmental Glomerulosclerosis. FSGS is a glomerular disease that disproportionately affects African Americans. It results in scarring of the glomerulus or clustering of glomeruli in a specific segment of the kidney. FSGS can be difficult to diagnose and treat. Biopsies to search for scarring in kidney tissue are the best means of a diagnosis. (A *biopsy* is a procedure in which a small amount of tissue is removed from the body for investigation and testing.) However, if the biopsy sample is from an unaffected area of the kidney, scarring will not be evident. Thus, repeated biopsies in different segments of the kidney are needed to confirm a diagnosis of FSGS.

The high prevalence of FSGS in African Americans has been traced to the gene *apolipoprotein L1, APOL1* for short.[39] The variants of this gene appear to have arisen in West Africa to combat parasites that cause African sleeping sickness. Moreover, these variants are not found in other racial groups. To make things worse, the rate of decline of kidney function is greater in those with high-risk variants of *APOL1* regardless of diabetes status. Finally, kidney transplants from deceased donors with high-risk variants of the *APOL1* gene shorten the survival times of kidney transplants.

FSGS can also develop in non–African Americans from genetic origins, which can involve up to forty genes, and nongenetic ones such as from exposure to viruses like HIV and certain medications.[40] The mechanisms of damage induced by FSGS are not completely understood but appear to involve injury to cells called *podocytes*, which help construct part of the kidney.

The body's immune system provides the first line of defense against infections by generating antibodies and immunoglobulins. However, there are times when antibodies and immunoglobulins cause harm to the body, which can lead to many medical problems. One of these complications is the deposit of antibodies in the glomeruli, causing inflammation.

Immunoglobulin A Nephropathy. Many autoimmune disorders contribute to glomerular diseases. One of these diseases is immunoglobulin A (IgA) nephropathy. (Immunoglobulin A is a class of antibodies with a particular structure.) IgA nephropathy is the most common cause of glomerular diseases not related to the presence of another disease. According to the National Institutes of Health, IgA nephropathy affects men twice as often as women, and in men it begins in their teens to late 30s. IgA nephropathy occurs more often in those with a family history of the disease and in people of either Asian or European descent. People with IgA nephropathy have an IgA with an abnormal structure that the immune system sees as foreign. The abnormal IgA and the other antibodies in the immune system that attack it form clumps, which

stick on the glomerulus, causing inflammation. Since a considerable amount of protein appears in the urine from this disease,
controlling blood pressure helps manage the symptoms and may
slow the rate of deterioration of kidney function. In addition, immunosuppressant drugs, such as steroids, can help to reduce the
inflammation.

Lupus Nephritis. Systemic lupus erythematosus (SLE), another
complex, multisymptomatic, autoimmune disease, primarily involves inflammation of the skin and joints as well as other organs.
SLE is found most often in North America and is lowest in Africa,
Ukraine, and North Australia in the limited populations studied.[41]
This disease affects women up to ten times more often than men,
according to the American College of Rheumatology, although
men are diagnosed at a more advanced age. When lupus attacks
the kidney, a condition known as lupus nephritis, autoantibodies
form or are deposited in the glomeruli, causing scarring. Genetic
as well as environmental factors also contribute to SLE.[42] Recently,
another possible mechanism has been suggested: imbalances in
intestinal composition of bacteria.[43] Although drugs that suppress
the immune system are generally used to treat the inflammation
in the kidney, correcting the bacterial imbalances may be a future
treatment option for lupus.

Alport's Syndrome. One inherited form of glomerular diseases
is Alport's syndrome. Alport's syndrome not only affects the kidney
but may also impair vision and hearing. More men have difficulty
with this disease than women, experiencing a decline in kidney
function in their twenties and reaching kidney failure by age 40.
According to the National Kidney Foundation, three genes underlie Alport's syndrome. Mutations of these genes alter the structure
and function of collagen, a protein important in healthy kidney
function. There is no cure for Alport's syndrome, but the loss of
kidney function can be reduced by treating high blood pressure
and limiting salt in the diet.

Finally, glomerular diseases are also caused by infections in other parts of the body. Like what happens in autoimmune diseases, the high number of antibodies produced to combat these infections can deposit in the kidneys and reduce kidney function. Although infections usually do not cause permanent damage, people with chronic infectious diseases such as HIV/AIDS and hepatitis C have an increased risk of developing CKD.

Polycystic Kidney Disease

Polycystic kidney disease (PKD), the fourth leading cause of CKD, accounts for about 5 percent of people with CKD. In PKD, small, fluid-filled cysts develop in the kidneys, sometimes even before birth. These cysts grow large enough over time to cause kidney failure. Because the cysts can grow so large, physicians used to think PKD was a form of kidney cancer.

According to the PKD Foundation, PKD affects 600,000 Americans and more than ten million people worldwide of both genders and all ethnic groups. PKD is the most common inherited kidney disease. Although it can occur spontaneously, most people inherit PKD. In fact, PKD is one of the most life-threatening inherited diseases. Because PKD is primarily inherited, research has identified the genes and their corresponding proteins responsible for the disease. As a result, understanding what these proteins do may lead to better treatments of PKD.

People with PKD inherit the disease from one or both of their parents, depending on the form of the disease. PKD comes in two forms: *autosomal dominant* (ADPKD), the more common form of the disease, and *autosomal recessive* (ARPKD). A thorough review of the genetics and mechanisms of PKD can be found elsewhere.[44]

Genetically, the difference between ADPKD and ARPKD is the number of faulty copies inherited (figures 3.8 and 3.9). People with ADPKD inherit the mutated gene from only one parent, whereas people with ARPKD inherit one mutated gene from both parents. The gene inherited in ARPKD is different from the one inherited in ADPKD.

FIGURE 3.8. Autosomal Dominant Inheritance of PKD (ADPKD)

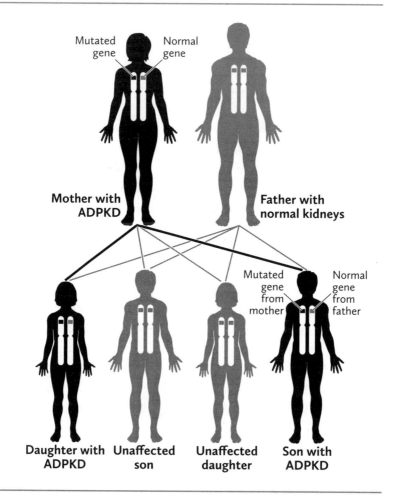

ADPKD is common, affecting 1 in 500 people. Because a person needs to inherit only one copy of an abnormal gene from one affected parent to get ADPKD, the chance of inheriting PKD when one parent has the defect is 50 percent. Because both parents must have the mutated gene, inheriting ARPKD is much less common, affecting 1 in 20,000 people in the general population. With ARPKD, if only one parent carries the mutated gene but does not

FIGURE 3.9. Autosomal Recessive Inheritance of PKD (ARPKD)

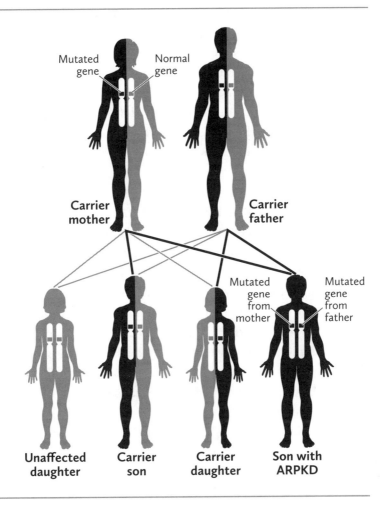

have the disease, offspring will not develop ARPKD but may pass on the mutated gene to their children. A person whose parents both have a mutated ARPKD gene has a 25 percent chance of inheriting the disease.

ADPKD and ARPKD also develop differently. The onset of ADPKD can occur at any age from the late teens to the midthirties, with CKD generally developing between the midforties and midfifties. Because the rate of cyst formation is variable, a person with ADPKD may not need dialysis until an advanced age. Sometimes ADPKD is diagnosed unexpectedly during a routine physical, where abnormal lab results suggest kidney disease. More tests would be needed for a definitive diagnosis (see below). ARPKD, in comparison, often progresses before birth. A person with ARPKD can only survive into adulthood with dialysis or transplantation. In this book, I use the terms ADPKD and PKD interchangeably, since the incidence of ARPKD is so low and will not be discussed further.

During the past twenty years, research has revealed the genetic underpinnings of PKD. Two genes, *PKD1* and *PKD2*, account for virtually all cases of PKD. Mutations in *PKD1* account for 80 percent of PKD cases. In most of the other cases of PKD, mutations in *PKD2* are responsible.

Although the disease caused by each mutated gene is similar, people with *PKD2* mutations tend to progress toward CKD later in life than people with *PKD1* mutations. In addition, people with *PKD2* mutations have fewer renal cysts when diagnosed and are less likely to have high blood pressure. People with *PKD1* mutations experience CKD earlier in life because they have more cysts than people with *PKD2* mutations.

Genes make proteins. *PKD1* and *PKD2* make the proteins polycystin-1 and polycystin-2, respectively, which play crucial roles in the growth of cysts. Research has shown that the two proteins are attached to one another. Although a mutation in the genes and improper working of the proteins are necessary for PKD to progress, other unknown factors may explain why the disease develops differently across families and even within families. A main factor is hypertension. If not treated adequately, high blood pressure promotes the growth of cysts and faster progression to kidney failure.

Our understanding of how renal cysts form and grow has progressed thanks to scientific research. Epithelial cells lining the tubules in the kidneys are actively involved in reabsorbing nutrients and water (see chapter 2). In PKD, about 1 percent of epithelial cells reproduce many times and eventually form numerous cysts. These cysts fill up with fluid and eventually press against the nephrons so that no urine can pass through them. When enough nephrons are blocked, the kidneys cease to function. The cysts that form in the kidneys can become quite large (figure 3.10). A normal kidney weighs less than a pound. A polycystic kidney can weigh up to thirty-eight pounds and may produce a protruding abdomen.

FIGURE 3.10. A Polycystic Kidney (*left*) Can Be Much Larger Than a Normal Kidney (*right*)

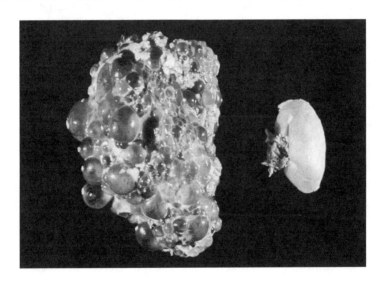

Source: PKD Foundation.

Experimental studies of the polycystins suggest that they determine the width of the tubules in the kidney. In effect, they tell the epithelial cells lining tubules when to stop growing. Tubular growth stops if they receive a signal from a messenger to do so. Although the nature of all the messengers and signals is unknown, presumably involving both polycystins, the epithelial cells must continue to receive the signal to stop growing, or they will continue to reproduce and develop into fluid-filled cysts.

One important discovery is that kidney epithelial cells possess hairlike structures called cilia that extend into the tubules. Like wheat bending in the wind, cilia bend in response to the movement of urine in the tubules. Cilia contain polycystin-1 and polycystin-2, suggesting a role for these structures in the development of cysts.

Polycystin-2 is associated with calcium movements, and a link between cilia and calcium-mediated cyst formation and PKD seems plausible. Indeed, the bending of cilia increases the inflow of calcium into epithelial cells. Perhaps in normal kidneys, the flow of urine deflects the cilia, thereby setting in motion a chain of calcium-mediated, biochemical reactions that place a lid on epithelial cell production. In the case of PKD kidneys, the cilia may not respond to deflection resulting in uncontrolled cell production and cysts.

Specific biochemical pathways have been identified that may be involved in cyst formation.[44] One of the most important is the discovery that the hormone *vasopressin* plays a significant role. Vasopressin when secreted from the pituitary gland causes the body to retain water and works through a mediator called *adenosine cyclic monophosphate* (cAMP).[45] Working through a receptor, this latter action supports cyst growth. This finding has led to the first treatment for PKD approved by the Food and Drug Administration: the drug tolvaptan blocks a vasopressin receptor, and that blocks cyst growth and promotes water loss (chapter 5).

Although the extent to which any of the mechanisms described significantly contributes to the development of PKD, the steps leading to cyst formation are becoming clearer. As we begin to understand the way mutations in the PKD genes occur and the underlying mechanisms of cyst formation, the knowledge obtained could lead to new strategies to prevent PKD from progressing to CKD.

Until recently, early diagnosis of PKD had been difficult, but now noninvasive techniques like ultrasound, computerized tomography (CT) scans, and magnetic resonance imaging (MRI) scans are used to identify renal cysts.[44] Ultrasound detects ADPKD in most people by 30 years of age. However, ultrasound may miss some cases involving the *PKD2* gene. CT scans produce clearer images but require exposure to radiation and contrast dyes.

A long-term study found that measuring increases in kidney size (cyst volume) using MRI scans is the best method of diagnosing and following the progression of PKD and is an excellent predictor of the loss of kidney function.[46] Using MRI scans to measure kidney size is not yet part of general clinical practice, but this approach could provide more precise measurements of disease progression and of the effectiveness of possible medical treatments.

One of the earliest problems found in people with PKD is high blood pressure. This can significantly increase the progression of the disease by activating the renin-angiotensin system.[47] Controlling blood pressure, especially with inhibitors of angiotensin converting enzyme, can retard the further progression of PKD. Since children with PKD can have high blood pressure, they should be monitored even if they have not been diagnosed but have a family history of PKD.[44]

Like diabetes, PKD can have numerous health consequences. Kidney cysts can be quite painful and may require surgery. People with PKD may have blood in the urine, frequent kidney infections, and urinary tract infections that require hospitalization. In some cases, the kidneys must be removed.

People with PKD may also have cysts form in the liver or other organs. The cysts can become large and uncomfortable, especially in women, requiring removal of part of the liver or drainage of the fluid in the cysts.

A potentially fatal complication of PKD is the ballooning (called an *aneurysm*) and rupture of a major blood vessel, especially in the brain.[44] Aneurysms occur in 5 to 10 percent of people with PKD and are five times greater than in the general population. Where a family history of aneurysms exists, the risk of aneurysm rises to nearly 30 percent. Modern imaging techniques can detect aneurysms by visualizing affected blood vessels, and people with PKD should be tested if they have a family history of aneurysms. If found early, aneurysms of a certain size can be repaired surgically. Small aneurysms are monitored with periodic scans. If scans show no aneurysms with a family history of aneurysms, repeated imaging at five-year intervals still may be warranted.[48]

Kidney Diseases in Children

Parents reading this book may be concerned about what causes CKD in children. According to the National Institutes of Health, such diseases can be grouped into several categories: birth defects, hereditary diseases, infections, nephrotic syndrome, and systemic diseases. These problems are generally rare. When such problems are seen depends on the age of a child. Between birth and age 4, birth defects and hereditary diseases most likely cause CKD. In children aged 5 to 14, kidney disease is most likely caused by hereditary, nephrotic, and systemic diseases. From age 15 to 19, diseases that cause kidney scarring are the most likely causes.

Children can be born with only one kidney, one that does not function, or one that is in the wrong place. Normally, children lead a normal life but are at risk of developing a kidney disease if the native one malfunctions or is damaged.

A couple of kidney diseases already discussed are hereditary and begin in childhood. Most notably, ARPKD and Alport's syndrome. Because these diseases require an affected gene from both parents, they are rare. Symptoms begin early in life and will likely result in the need for kidney replacement, either from dialysis or transplantation.

In a few cases, infections can lead to CKD. These infections are bacterial, and one cause is food poisoning. Contaminated foods can destroy red blood cells and the walls of blood vessels, including those in the glomerulus, leading to scarring. Another type of infection related to strep throat can induce a buildup of antibodies that can attack the kidneys. Usually, kidney problems are short lived, but, in some cases, damage can be permanent.

Nephrotic syndrome is a collection of symptoms, including blood in the urine, high levels of blood lipids, and fluid retention in the legs, ankles, and feet. The cause of this syndrome in children is not clear, but the results can be similar to infections: kidney scarring and a buildup of antibodies.

Finally, systemic diseases include lupus nephritis and diabetes. Although these diseases are not seen in a large population of children, concern is rising because of the rise in obesity. In general, the prevalence of CKD in children is still low, so perhaps these diseases can be contained.

Environmental Causes of Chronic Kidney Disease

Besides the conditions just described that can lead to CKD, there are many other less frequent medical and nonmedical causes. From our preceding discussion, it shouldn't be surprising that many environmental factors can cause CKD. Eating high quantities of salt and sugar come to mind, which can lead to hypertension or diabetes. But there are substances that we don't normally think of that might damage our kidneys. According to the National Kidney Foundation, these substances fall into three categories: (1) medications, (2) legal and illegal drugs, and (3) contrast dyes used in medical imaging, such as CT and MRI scans.

Medications for relieving pain, such as aspirin, ibuprofen, and naproxen, also known as nonsteroidal anti-inflammatory drugs (NSAIDS), have been shown to damage kidneys, especially with high doses and prolonged use. Those with CKD must be particularly careful in using these medications. However, pain is often associated with CKD, especially in those suffering from PKD. With the threat of addiction to opiates, NSAIDS might be useful in select patients for pain management.[49] As a result, it is best to use them only under supervision by your doctor.

Several legal and illegal drugs can have direct or indirect effects on the kidney. Of the legal ones, smoking and alcohol consumption can adversely affect the kidneys. This occurs predominately by worsening existing problems, such as high blood pressure and diabetes.[50] Smoking can raise blood pressure and interfere with the medications used to treat hypertension.

According to the National Kidney Foundation, the drying effect of high alcohol consumption can compromise the normal function of kidneys and raise blood pressure. However, recent research suggests that moderate alcohol consumption (two drinks per day for men, one drink per day for women) may lower the risk of CKD and diabetes.[51] I am not advocating that you start drinking alcohol for these possible benefits. The margin between benefits and toxic effects of alcohol is too narrow. There are other, better ways to reduce risk for CKD (chapter 5).

Illegal and semilegal drugs can have adverse effects on those with CKD. Although marijuana has been used to reduce side effects of CKD,[52] synthetic marijuana, under such names as Spice, K2, herbal incense, Cloud 9, and Mojo, should be avoided because they have been reported to produce serious kidney damage.[53] Other illegal drugs, such as heroin, cocaine, amphetamines, and ecstasy, raise blood pressure and can damage the kidneys.

Finally, contrast dyes used in CT and MRI scans can be problematic in those with CKD. They can cause acute kidney damage, especially with gadolinium-based dyes. Although kidney damage is rare, those with CKD should consult their health care team about whether the dye should be used.

Finally, reports over the past decade of CKD developing among agricultural workers in Central America has raised alarm in medical circles.[54] It is seen mostly in men who work as cane cutters on sugarcane plantations. As a result of their inability to pay for treatment, many of them die of kidney failure. This problem is not confined to Central America. Reports of CKD in agriculture workers in California, Florida, India, and Sri Lanka have surfaced. The cause of this problem is not completely known but probably involves a combination of heat stress, dehydration, and mineral loss. Hydration with minerals may have some benefit, but that has not yet been established.

Genetic Tests

Because genetic influences contribute to all four of the causes of kidney failure we have discussed, can tests identify people who are (or whose descendants are) at risk of developing kidney disease? Would a test help these people modify their lifestyle to reduce their chances of getting kidney disease or developing kidney failure? Perhaps. Some genetic tests can find the genes that cause diseases like diabetes. But because so many genes can contribute to each disease, it is not clear at this time how valuable such tests would be. Some gene data companies, such as 23andMe, sell such tests for a variety of diseases, but people should be cautious when using them and consult their health care team and a genetic counselor if they obtain any positive results. In addition, genetic testing may be available in research studies. Genetic testing generally is not covered by insurance and may have more value in predicting the progression of a disease rather than diagnosing one.

Testing for PKD can be useful because the genes for the disease have been identified. A genetic test has been developed by Athena Diagnostics (www.athenadiagnostics.com) to sequence *PKD1* and *PKD2* and to look for mutations. The test is effective only 70 percent of the time, however, so the results are possibly misleading. Sometimes the results give a false positive for the presence of PKD. Conversely, the results can miss actual cases of PKD. Testing in research labs that have more advanced genetic tests may give better results. Results of these genetic tests should be confirmed by an ultrasound.[55]

Genetic testing for PKD or other diseases may have some advantages. For those who want to know if they have the disease, it can give them peace of mind one way or another and allow them to plan for the future. Perhaps more importantly, clinical research has suggested that the time to intervene might be early in the progression of the disease. Genetic testing and/or imaging studies, therefore, might be worth considering.

Although genetic testing has its advantages, there are disadvantages that might deter some people from being tested. One drawback of finding out you have a disease is the emotional burden that knowledge brings with it. Since there is little you can do about having a disease such as PKD, other than good medical management for symptoms like hypertension and drinking a lot of fluid, what purpose would be served by knowing? Another drawback: a diagnosis of PKD may make it difficult to obtain medical and life insurance. If you do not have continuous employment, a new employer may not provide adequate insurance. If you are unemployed, you may not be able to obtain insurance at all. Having a definitive diagnosis of PKD may not be useful until signs of CKD or other symptoms like hypertension or kidney cysts appear. Legislation to bar genetic discrimination in obtaining medical insurance and employment was signed into federal law with the Genetic Information Non-Discrimination Act (GINDA) of 2008. In addition, Congress passed the Patient Protection and Affordable Care Act in 2010 that prohibits excluding people with preexisting conditions from obtaining health insurance. Currently, this legislation is being challenged in the courts and is in danger of being overturned. If so, the GINDA is still on the books but may require litigation to enforce it.

People with PKD may have trouble deciding whether to have children. Although children have a fifty-fifty chance of *not* inheriting a PKD mutated gene from an affected parent, they also have a fifty-fifty chance that they *do* have one. These odds are high enough to give some people pause before deciding to start a family. Parents can take solace in the hope that a cure might emerge for their children with PKD. In my own family, my mother died prematurely at age 44, when dialysis and transplantation were not available. I am in my seventies, and I have survived with a successful kidney transplant and am living a normal life. Today's medicine can treat CKD, anemia, high blood pressure, and other complicating factors of the disease. In my mother's day, none of these treatments existed. Tomorrow's medicine may be much more advanced, and a treatment to prevent cyst formation or growth may be available, relieving our children of the burden of PKD. Indeed, tolvaptan has been approved as the first medication to treat PKD (chapter 5).

There is hope for better treatment options in the future.

CHAPTER 4

Diagnosing and Managing Chronic Kidney Disease

A SIGNIFICANT NUMBER of people do not know they have kidney disease until they are in late stages. At particularly high risk are people over 60 years old; who have type 2 diabetes and cardiovascular disease, especially high blood pressure; who have a family history of kidney disease, particularly PKD; and who are in certain ethnic groups. These groups include African Americans, Native Americans, Hispanics, and Pacific Islanders (chapter 1). Thus, these high-risk groups should be screened regularly.

For everyone else, discovering chronic kidney disease (CKD) may happen during a routine checkup when your doctor finds a risk for CKD or that you already have CKD. Although it usually has no symptoms, such as fatigue or pain, at least at early stages, a physical examination can determine whether diabetes, high blood pressure, blood in the urine, or other causes have resulted in decreased kidney function. A thorough medical history will help your doctor know whether you have a predisposition to kidney disease or a family history of diseases that can lead to kidney disease, again like diabetes, high blood pressure, or polycystic kidney disease (PKD).

If you have one or more of these risk factors, your doctor may order additional screening tests. The National Kidney Foundation (NKF) has developed a screening program for risk of developing CKD called the Kidney Early Evaluation Program (KEEP). Your doctor may use certain measures to assess your risk and to find any evidence of CKD and whether it has progressed. The measures of assessing risk are listed in table 4.1. Screening typically consists of *urinalysis* (looking for protein or blood in the urine) and measuring creatinine or other factors in the blood. With a measure of blood creatinine, your doctor will calculate your glomerular filtration rate, a measure of the ability of your kidneys to filter toxins from your blood. The results of these tests may cause your doctor to suspect that you have kidney disease. A definite plus is that the results of the tests may provide an early warning, so your doctor can help you protect your kidneys from further damage and educate

TABLE 4.1 Kidney Early Evaluation Program (KEEP) Screening Measures

Measures	Significance
↑ Blood pressure	Risk of kidney disease
Height, weight, and waist circumference	Obesity; risk of diabetes and kidney disease
↑ Blood glucose	Risk of diabetes
↓ Hemoglobin	Anemia
White blood cells in urine	Risk for infections, inflammation, and other abnormalities in the urinary tract
Red blood cells in the urine	Evidence of kidney disease
Protein in the urine	Evidence of kidney disease
↓ Glomerular filtration rate	Evidence of kidney failure
↑ Total cholesterol, ↓ HDL, ↑ LDL, and ↑ triglycerides	Risk for cardiovascular disease
↓ Calcium, ↑ phosphorus, ↑ parathyroid hormone	Evidence of possible bone disease

Source: Adapted from the list of KEEP measures from National Kidney Foundation website at www.kidney.org.

you about treatment options or changes in lifestyle. For example, your doctor may recommend that you lose weight, stop smoking, or control your blood pressure.

Being diagnosed with any disease can be terrifying. If you are diagnosed with CKD, gather as much information as you can about your condition and medical care, find ways to reduce the progression of CKD, and plan your future. Take an active role in your care. It will go a long way toward helping you feel more in control. This chapter covers some of the diagnostic tools and treatments involved with your medical care.

Diagnostics

Doctors monitor kidney function in their patients by measuring substances in the blood and urine using several laboratory tests: blood urea nitrogen (BUN), or just urea, creatinine, creatinine clearance, glomerular filtration rate (GFR), and urinary protein. To perform these tests, your health care provider will draw small amounts of blood and will ask you for a urine sample.

Urea and creatinine in the blood are measures of the main products of protein breakdown. How concentrated these substances are in the blood indicates how effectively your kidneys remove waste products. Normal concentrations of these substances are 15 to 25 mg/dL for BUN and 0.5 to 1.3 mg/dL for creatinine (mg/dL [milligrams per deciliter] refers to the amount of a substance in a bit more than 3 ounces of blood). Depending on the laboratory in which the analysis is performed, normal values may be different. Otherwise, values higher than that range for either measurement mean that kidney function is declining.

A *blood urea nitrogen* (BUN) test measures the quantity of nitrogen in your blood that comes from the waste product urea. A BUN is performed to see how well your kidneys are functioning. If your kidneys can't remove urea from the blood, your BUN level will rise.

Measuring *creatinine clearance* can determine how much creatinine your kidneys remove from your body as well as how well your kidneys are functioning. Creatinine clearance is a more precise measure of kidney function than relying on blood measurements alone. To perform a creatinine clearance test, your doctor will ask you to collect your urine over a twenty-four-hour period in a large container. A laboratory will then analyze your urine for creatinine. In addition to a urinalysis, a small amount of your blood will be analyzed for creatinine. Your calculated creatinine clearance is expressed as the volume of blood your kidneys completely clear of creatinine per minute. A normal creatinine clearance ranges from 90 to 130 mL/min (milliliter per minute). As kidney function declines, creatinine clearance also drops.

Glomerular filtration rate (GFR), the preferred method for assessing kidney function, is a test similar to creatinine clearance. Your doctor or a laboratory can estimate GFR from blood creatinine—considering age, gender, race, and body mass—using the GFR calculator provided by the NKF (http://www.kidney.org/professionals/kdoqi/gfr_calculator.cfm; or go to www.kidney.org and click on "Kidney Professionals" and then on "eGFR Calculator" under "Tools & resources"). Like creatinine clearance, GFR provides more accurate information about kidney function than blood creatinine alone does. Normal values are 80 to 120 mL/min./1.73 m². From the value obtained, your doctor can determine the stage of CKD and can easily monitor its progression without having to obtain a twenty-four-hour urine collection from you each time your blood creatinine is measured. In addition, she can use this information to plan your treatment. Several measures of GFR are available, but the one most preferred is the GFR-EPI. It considers your blood creatinine level, age, gender, and race (African American or not).

Under some circumstances, the GFR may not give a clear indication of kidney function. Those who are obese, elderly, or highly muscular, such as body builders, might fall into this situation. With the obese, body surface area can be underestimated. With age,

GFR could be overstated. With highly muscular people, natural creatinine levels could be high enough to suggest kidney disease when there is none. To circumvent this problem, your doctor could order a measurement of cystatin C, a protein in cells that the kidneys keep at a stable level. When kidney function declines, cystatin C levels will rise. So, this test can be used by your doctor as a supplement if he feels that the GFR is not giving an accurate measure of kidney function.

Once CKD has been revealed through one of the tests described earlier, your doctor may refer you to a nephrologist. The NKF's guidelines suggest that patients be referred to a nephrologist when their GFR is less than 30. Your doctor may also refer you to a nephrologist at higher GFRs, if you have blood in your urine, a rapid and unexplained drop in kidney function, an inherited kidney disease, difficult-to-treat high blood pressure, or unexplained electrolyte imbalances. In addition, you may be referred to a nephrologist if protein in the urine is abnormally high, even though you may still be in an early stage of CKD.[1]

The stages of CKD are displayed in table 4.2.[2] Stage G1 is defined as the stage when GFR is 90 or higher, but there are markers of kidney damage, such as protein in the urine or kidney cysts in people who have PKD. Your doctor will check your heart's health and will look for any other cardiovascular issues. At stage G1 your doctor will concentrate on finding the cause of your kidney disease and on treating any underlying disease, such as diabetes and high blood pressure.

Stage G2 is classified by a GFR of 60 to 89. In addition to giving you a diagnosis of your stage, and treating you, your doctor will try to slow the decline of your kidney function, perhaps prescribing medications to control your blood pressure, to lower elevated blood sugar, or to help treat other underlying diseases. *During stages G1 and G2, you must follow your doctor's recommendations, even if you don't feel sick.* By doing so, you have the greatest chance of postponing the complete loss of kidney function, perhaps indefinitely. In addition, you may have no symptoms of kidney disease and you may feel well enough to live a normal life.

At stages G3a and G3b, with a GFR of 30 to 59, there are more evident complications of CKD. For example, you may become anemic (loss of red blood cells), show evidence of bone disease, or have a poor nutritional status. A poor nutritional status might be caused in part by an impaired smelling ability.[3] Although it may be years before your kidneys completely fail, if at all, your nephrologist may introduce you to future treatment options for CKD, including dialysis and transplantation. This discussion is especially relevant for younger patients. This is also a time when people start feeling ill for the first time, in many cases not knowing that they had CKD.

TABLE 4.2 GFR Categories in CKD

GFR Category	GFR (mL/min./1.73 m²)	Terms
G1	≥90	Normal or high
G2	60–89	Mildly decreased
G3a	45–59	Mildly to moderately decreased
G3b	30–44	Moderately to severely decreased
G4	15–29	Severely decreased
G5	<15	Kidney failure

If you reach stage G4, with a GFR of 15 to 29, your nephrologist may prepare you for dialysis by explaining the process and may have you evaluated for a kidney transplant (chapters 6 and 7). He will explain the drawbacks and benefits of these treatments and help you decide which one is best for you and your lifestyle. It's a painful fact that a transplant may not be available for years, if you don't have a donor. Your doctor can help you plan how to integrate these treatments into your life to make them as unobtrusive as possible.

Stage G5, when GFR is less than 15, means that you probably need dialysis or transplantation to live. Exactly when this happens is subject to Medicare rules and medical judgment. To be referred for dialysis, your GFR must be <15, although for transplantation, you can be referred with a GFR <20 but transplanted when GFR <15. Even these are not the only reasons to start dialysis or to have a transplant. For example, those with untreatable fluid retention, high blood potassium, or acidosis may qualify for early dialysis or transplantation. In other cases, however, when patients are frail, have other concurring medical problems, or choose to decline dialysis, supportive care often is a better option than dialysis. Supportive options emphasize providing comfort and maximizing the quality of life.[4]

Serum creatinine levels are a useful gauge of kidney function, but by themselves, they are not a reliable indication of disease. Assessing the degree of kidney decline solely from these levels can be misleading. When serum creatinine levels are followed over time, they may appear to rise rapidly. However, calculating the GFRs for these values can provide a different picture. Changes in serum creatinine from stage 1 to 2 in the normal range represent much larger percentage changes in GFR than when they rise from stage 3 to 4. While on the surface it would seem that a change in the higher levels (stages 3 and 4) would cause more concern than an increase from stage 1 to 2, we have to consider that a 100 percent change (from stage 1 to 2) is larger than a 33 percent change (from stage 3 to 4). It could be many years before you will need dialysis or transplantation, if at all. Thus, it is not that kidney function has declined faster, it just seems that way because you are only looking at creatinine, not GFR. In other words, your kidney function is not declining as fast as you may fear it is.

Your doctor will also determine whether you are anemic (chapter 2). Red blood cells, hemoglobin, and hematocrit are all factors in diagnosing anemia. *Hemoglobin* is a protein in red blood cells that carries oxygen from the lungs to the rest of the body. Normal hemoglobin concentrations are between 14.0 g/dL and 18.0 g/dL (grams per deciliter). *Hematocrit* measures the percentage of blood volume occupied by red blood cells. Normal hematocrit values are 40 to 54 percent for men and 37 to 47 percent for women. Low hemoglobin or hematocrit values may mean you have anemia, a condition that is common in more advanced stages of kidney disease.

Your Nephrologist

If you are happy with your primary care doctor, then her recommended nephrologist will probably be someone you will come to trust as well. But personal interactions are subjective, and different patients may view the same doctor differently, for all kinds of reasons. If you sense that you are not getting the nephrologist's full attention; if the nephrologist will not explain terms, concepts, or recommended medical care; or if you feel that your condition is not properly managed, you may want to consider getting a second opinion from another nephrologist. It may be that you will want to switch doctors, or the second opinion may reinforce your confidence in your current nephrologist.

Once you have been referred to a nephrologist, he will become an important member of your medical team, although your family physician will continue providing your general care. Your nephrologist may be one of several doctors involved in your health care, depending on the underlying disease causing your CKD. For example, if you have heart disease, a cardiologist may be monitoring your cardiac health; if you have diabetes, an endocrinologist may be managing your blood sugar; if you have lupus, a rheumatologist may be treating inflammation. Ideally, all your doctors will work together as a team and will communicate closely with you and with one another.

The stage and the cause of CKD determine the recommended treatment. Many people do not see a nephrologist until their kidney disease is fairly advanced, because they do not know they have CKD until it reaches a later stage. But if you do see a nephrologist at an early stage, he can focus on the underlying cause and possibly intervene to reduce the progression of CKD as well as manage any signs and symptoms you may have.

A first visit to the nephrologist will include a thorough examination of your medical records, as well as assessments of your kidney function, urine, or any diagnosed kidney disease. If you have no diagnosed disease, your nephrologist will begin by identifying the primary cause of your declining kidney function. In addition, if the nephrologist has ruled out acute or short-term kidney failure, she will want to know your stage of CKD. With a diagnosis, the nephrologist can work to decrease the rate of loss of kidney function, to control your blood pressure, and, depending on the stage of CKD, to manage any complications. (Complications typically begin when your GFR is below 60.) Your nephrologist may also recommend an ultrasound of your kidneys to measure their size or to locate cysts or stones. A kidney biopsy may be necessary to make a diagnosis and to help determine the best way to treat you.

Ask your nephrologist any questions you have about your disease. She should help you understand CKD and your long-term prognosis. She can also educate you about new treatments and the latest research that may ultimately lead to slowing the progression of kidney disease.

The information your nephrologist shares with you during your first visit depends on the underlying cause of your kidney disease. If you have diabetes and excrete protein in your urine, your nephrologist will advise you to control your blood sugar and blood pressure with diet and medications. If applicable, your nephrologist will recommend that you lose weight, stop smoking, and take measures to lower your cholesterol.

If you have PKD, you may be newly diagnosed and in the early stages of the disease, with only a few cysts in your kidneys. It could be many years before there is a need for dialysis or transplantation. Moreover, if you are newly diagnosed and older than 50, you may never need dialysis or transplantation, especially if you have only a few cysts. The discussion of dialysis and transplantation varies greatly, depending on many factors.

By stage G3, however, you may have lost half of your kidney function. At that point, your nephrologist may advise you that you may need dialysis or a transplant in the future.

It is important that you understand the difference between *stability* of kidney function and *level* of kidney function. For example, your nephrologist may be satisfied if your creatinine remains at 3.0. However, he might not always remind you that you have lost more than half of your kidney function, and that being stable with poor kidney function is not normal. GFR almost never improves. Remember, your nephrologist wants to be reassuring while he wants you to take care of yourself. If it has been a while since you discussed your prognosis with your nephrologist, ask him to discuss your future with you.

Managing the Consequences of Chronic Kidney Disease

As you read earlier in this chapter, you may encounter several consequences involving other organs and processes in your body as your kidney function declines. Although these problems can be worrisome, your nephrologist can help you manage them.

Kidney disease is a primary risk factor for heart disease—including heart attacks—as are smoking and high cholesterol. As a result, your nephrologist will encourage you to manage your blood pressure and to live a healthy lifestyle. Living a healthy lifestyle is one aspect of your care over which you have total control. You can manage your diet more than almost any other aspect of your life.

As your kidneys lose their ability to work properly, eating a heart-healthy diet is essential—along with managing your blood pressure and lowering your cholesterol. If you are obese, lose weight and begin an exercise program. If you smoke tobacco, stop smoking. Get help with weight loss and smoking cessation if needed.

Depending on the stage of CKD, your nephrologist may recommend that you eat a low-salt diet, especially if you have high blood pressure. Failing kidneys cannot eliminate the excess salt consumed, and so the soft tissues of the body begin to accumulate fluid. This accumulated fluid, called *edema*, can be uncomfortable, especially if it collects in the legs and ankles. Fluid accumulating in the lungs restricts the airway and can impair breathing. Prescription diuretics (water pills) can help control your edema if you can still pass adequate amounts of urine. Occasionally, excessive fluid in the lungs is a medical emergency, requiring hospitalization for removal. Tell your doctor immediately if you have any trouble breathing.

Your nephrologist might recommend a modest restriction of protein in your diet, because a lower-protein diet may slow the progression of kidney disease, especially if you have protein in your urine. You should eat a heart-healthy, high-fiber, low-fat, low-cholesterol diet. You can find more information about diet in chapter 5.

As we learned in chapter 2, kidneys do more than just filter waste products out of the blood. Kidneys also control blood pressure, regulate red blood cell production, maintain the proper acidity in the blood, control potassium and phosphate levels, and activate vitamin D to help build and maintain strong bones. When kidney function deteriorates, complications with these functions may arise and may require medical treatment.

Anemia

Low levels of red blood cells, or anemia, is one complication of CKD. Anemia can make people feel tired even with adequate sleep, have little energy, and have trouble thinking clearly. This problem is most likely experienced in later stages of CKD (stages 3–5), by

African Americans, by people with diabetes, and by women. As kidney function declines, the amount of the hormone erythropoietin available to regulate red blood cell production decreases, leading to anemia. Injectable synthetic hormone treatments such as Epogen (EPO), Procrit, or Aranesp (darbepoetin) may help treat anemia. A health care provider can inject the medication for you or teach you how to do it yourself.

Prescription hormone treatment for anemia is most effective for people with hemoglobin levels below 13 g/dL for men and 11 g/dL for women.[5] However, if hemoglobin levels become too high, hormone treatment may be unsafe, potentially causing higher blood pressure, heart problems, and blood clots. Your nephrologist will carefully monitor your hemoglobin to determine whether hormone treatment is right for you.

Blood Acidity

When kidneys can no longer regulate blood acidity, acid builds up, causing acidosis. If left untreated, acidosis can become a serious condition. It can even accelerate the decline in your kidney function.[6] If you have acidosis, your nephrologist will prescribe sodium bicarbonate (baking soda), which neutralizes the excess acid. You can use either regular baking soda that you find in the grocery store, sodium bicarbonate tablets, or sodium citrate liquid, which the body converts into bicarbonate. The important point here is getting treatment early may retard the progression of CKD.

High Potassium

Potassium levels in the blood may rise with progressing CKD. High potassium levels typically occur at stages 3–5. Normal kidneys regulate the amount of *potassium* in the blood by excreting excess potassium. As kidney function declines, however, the kidneys may lose this ability and blood potassium can increase, sometimes to dangerous levels. If high enough, potassium can disturb the heart's rhythm, increasing the chances of death.[7,8] High potassium is seen most often in people with low kidney function, with diabetes, and who take drugs to lower blood pressure through the angiotensin system (chapters 2 and 5).

If high blood potassium happens to you, you can help lower it by managing your diet. But, in some cases, your doctor may need to prescribe medications, such as patiromer (Veltassa), the older drug sodium polystyrene sulfonate (Kayexalate), or a diuretic such as furosemide (Lasix) to treat excess potassium. A dietitian can help you choose the right kinds of foods to avoid high potassium levels (tables 7.1 and 7.2 for high and low potassium foods, respectively). Your nephrologist will recommend a consultation with a dietitian if needed. Most dialysis centers have dietitians available.

High Phosphate

Phosphorus in the form of phosphate is important in the production of energy from consumed food. However, the body does not use all the phosphate ingested and must remove the excess amounts. Normally, the kidneys do that job. As kidney function deteriorates, however, the kidney cannot eliminate the excess phosphate, so it accumulates in the blood and binds to calcium, lowering calcium in the blood. In people on or nearing the start of dialysis (chapters 2 and 6), these deposits can, in the extreme, remove calcium from the bones and lead to bone disorders. People with high phosphorus may also experience itching. Therefore, people with high phosphorus levels must reduce phosphate intake (chapter 6) and may need to take medications to bind ingested phosphate before it can be absorbed. Over-the-counter calcium carbonate tablets like Tums or prescribed drugs like calcium acetate (PhosLo) and sevelamer (Renagel) can help control high phosphorus levels (tables 6.3 and 6.4 for high and low phosphate foods, respectively).

Low Vitamin D

As you lose kidney function, your body may not make enough kidney-activated vitamin D to maintain sufficient calcium levels to keep your bones strong. In addition, *parathyroid hormone* levels can rise, leaching calcium out of your bones. Parathyroid hormone is released from the parathyroid glands, located near the thyroid gland in your neck. In reverse to what happens with *excess* phosphate in the blood, *inadequate* levels of calcium can make your bones brittle, causing them to break more easily or begin to hurt. Your nephrologist can treat vitamin D deficiency with several drugs, such as paricalcitol (Zemplar) or calcitriol (Rocaltrol), synthetic forms that bypass the need for your kidneys to activate inactive forms of vitamin D (chapter 2).

Gout

Gout is an inflammatory, arthritic disorder resulting from a buildup of blood uric acid (called *hyperuricemia*), a normal waste product from the breakdown of purines. They are found in the body and many foods, such as red meat, some seafood (shrimp and lobster), liquor and beer, and sugar-sweetened products containing high-fructose corn syrup.

When blood uric acid rises, crystals can form and deposit themselves in the joints causing pain, swelling, stiffness, and deformity. Movement can also be impaired. In addition, the crystals can form large stones in the kidneys causing pain and possibly kidney damage. Ultimately, this damage can impair the removal of waste products and lead to scarring and a reduction in kidney function.

A complex relationship exists among gout, CKD, and several of its causes. Up to more than 30 percent of those with CKD have gout, depending on the stage of functional decline and age. As CKD progresses, the percentage of those with gout increases, with the highest percentage at stage 4 and in the elderly.[9,10] Gout enhances the chance of death in those with CKD by almost 80 percent.[11] On the flip side, those with only gout have a 57 percent higher risk of developing CKD, especially those over age 45.[12] Moreover, many of the diseases that cause or contribute to CKD, such as type 2 diabetes, high blood pressure, metabolic syndrome, and obesity, also worsen gout.[13] Thus, the interaction between these diseases and gout may have reinforcing effects on one another, increasing the number of gout attacks and the rate of decline of kidney function.

Fortunately, there is good news in the options available to treat gout. If you think you may be developing gout, consult your doctor to get tested and to see what medications would be best for you. The most common drugs are allopurinol (Aloprim, Zyloprim) and febuxostat (Uloric).[14] Some of the drugs available can damage your kidneys, so care must be taken to avoid further complicating your medical condition. In addition, modify your diet to restrict those foods most likely to worsen gout (such as the ones listed in the beginning of this section).

Depression

As mentioned in chapter 1, depression is one of a series of responses that people with CKD may experience to their CKD diagnosis. Although mild depression might not cause alarm, more severe and long-lasting depression can be dangerous. In fact, 20 to 40 percent of those with CKD experience depression, depending on the stage of the disease and the measure used for diagnosing depression.[15,16] In addition, depression can even increase the progression of CKD. Sometimes, depression is underdiagnosed, because some symptoms of CKD, for example, fatigue and sleep difficulties, might mask symptoms of depression.

Feeling a bit low on some days is normal, but if you feel that your mood is bad all the time or your family shows concern that you might be depressed, don't be afraid to ask for help. According to the American Kidney Fund, here are a few signs to look for that might suggest that you are depressed: difficulty sleeping, feeling more dependent on others than usual, feeling powerless to control your disease and its treatment, and pressure from friends and family to act in a manner inconsistent with your proper medical needs. This might include not following your kidney-friendly dietary needs when out with friends. Another cause of depression may be worry over medical costs and how they will be paid.[17] While Medicare may pay some costs for those who are eligible, for many low- and some middle-income people private insurance is either not available or too expensive. Inadequate access to health care can also contribute to depression.

If you are depressed, talk to your doctor about ways to cope with the problem. Treatment may include medications or behavioral techniques to help you cope with those aspects of life that contribute to your depression. Getting adequate sleep and exercise can go a long way to improve your mood. Finally, believe that you will get better and take control of your medical and personal life as much as possible. Looking forward to better times can improve your mood. The problems associated with CKD can be complicated and sometimes bewildering. Working with your doctor and your support group can help you work through the initial stages of recovery from depression, but recovery can take time. Don't expect improvement to come too quickly. Relapses can happen. Be patient and diligent and you should be okay.

The Signs and Symptoms of Failing Kidneys

When our kidneys are working normally, we may be unaware of their great ability to cleanse our bodies of the toxins that accumulate after we digest our food. Urination is the only overt sign that our kidneys work at all. And when our kidneys slowly begin to fail, we can detect, at first, only subtle changes in how we feel. Here are a few of my experiences with CKD and a description of how my nephrologist helped me.

During the first three stages of kidney disease, I felt fine. The only health issue I faced during that period was high blood pressure and a kidney infection. My first symptom of CKD was fatigue. My fatigue occurred slowly, so initially I didn't notice anything unusual. I just assumed I was working too hard or wasn't getting enough sleep. In time, fatigue became noticeable. By this point, I had reached stage G4 kidney disease.

During the two or three years before I began dialysis, I was so tired that I had difficulty getting up for work every morning, no matter how much sleep I got. Finally, after telling my nephrologist about my fatigue, tests showed that I had become very anemic. With fewer red blood cells carrying oxygen throughout my body, my muscles could no longer do what they needed to do for very long without my feeling debilitated.

My red blood cell count was very low, because I had lost so much of my own erythropoietin (EPO). As a result, my nephrologist prescribed an injectable form of the hormone to produce more red blood cells. Injecting it into my own body was similar to what people with diabetes do—injecting themselves with insulin to normalize their blood sugar. With practice, I found it easy to inject myself with EPO. Besides, I had to do it only once a week, rather than the twice-a-day injections of insulin. After several weeks of injections, I started feeling normal again. In the end, the fatigue I experienced confirmed what my increasing creatinine levels were already telling me: my kidneys were failing, and dialysis or transplantation was inevitable.

A year later, my fatigue returned, and I began to feel increasingly nauseated and was vomiting frequently. By then, I was approaching stage G5. Nausea and vomiting were the worst symptoms that I had. To help, my doctor prescribed ondansetron (Zofran), which is used to treat nausea and vomiting in people with cancer who are receiving chemotherapy or radiation treatments. Even this heavy-duty drug could not completely treat my symptoms. I had to tough it out until I could start dialysis or receive a transplant.

In addition to nausea and vomiting, I needed more EPO to keep my anemia under control. Moreover, I required additional medication to control my blood pressure. All this attention to treatment combined with symptoms sapped my energy, making it difficult for me to do anything. As my CKD accelerated, I had to decide, with the help of my nephrologist, when I would start dialysis, because I didn't have a kidney donor.

The decision whether to start dialysis or to receive a kidney transplant, if a donor kidney is available, is both a medical and a personal decision. Medically, people usually cannot start dialysis until their GFR is below 15. Generally, Medicare will not pay for dialysis or transplantation until GFR is 15 or less, except when your doctor has documented other reasons, like fluid overload, high potassium, or acidosis that cannot be corrected with fluid restriction or medications.

For me, the decision to start dialysis depended mostly on how bad I felt and on knowing that dialysis would require a significant change in my lifestyle. I talked to some people who thought they had waited too long. Although it can take some time, many people feel better after starting dialysis. The decision to get a transplant is usually an easy one, unless you are not medically fit for one. When my kidneys failed, I really had no choice. I had to do something, if I wanted to continue living. When I finally faced that decision, I started dialysis. As it turned out, it was not the end of the world. It saved my life.

I do not tell my story to scare you but to underscore the many ways to minimize the consequences of CKD. You should learn how to prevent or slow the progression of your declining kidney function. This knowledge can extend your healthy time before you must make life-altering decisions about dialysis or transplantation. Chapter 5 explores the various ways you can change your behavior, and chapter 6 looks at the various treatments to keep your kidneys working as long as possible.

CHAPTER 5

Preventing, Postponing, and Treating Chronic Kidney Disease

BENJAMIN FRANKLIN WROTE that an "ounce of prevention is worth a pound of cure." This adage is certainly true with chronic kidney disease (CKD). In chapter 3 we learned that the major causes of CKD—diabetes and hypertension—can be prevented. Even an inherited disease like polycystic kidney disease (PKD) has environmental and lifestyle components, where interventions can sometimes extend kidney function indefinitely in some cases. Who would not want to prevent their kidneys from failing? Certainly, few of us would intentionally live our lives in a way that might cause CKD. Many otherwise rational people, however, find it hard to do what is best for their health rather than what they are used to doing—or what they would prefer to do. Beyond human nature, there are several other factors that might circumvent early interventions that might prevent or delay CKD.

One of them is not knowing that you are sick. When we are young and healthy, it's easy to neglect our health. Most young people have no medical problems they know about, even though they may be vaguely aware of some that may lurk in the background. That was true for me in my late twenties. After I earned my doctorate, I pursued a research career as a visiting fellow at the National Institutes of Health. My fellowship did not provide health insurance, and I could not afford to buy it. Because I was healthy at the time and did not know I had PKD, I took the chance of doing without health insurance for my two-year fellowship. As a young man I thought I was invincible—that is, until I developed hypertension in my thirties. Even then, I took prescribed medications and went on with my life.

Even when the warning signs of impending disease appear, it can still be difficult to believe that we may eventually face a serious health condition like CKD. Denial may prevent us from taking immediate action for our medical condition, especially if we assume that the condition is not serious or that we have plenty of time to address it (chapter 1). Most people would prefer to focus their attention on more immediate issues. Often it takes a medical crisis to wake us up.

If we accept that we are at risk of a serious medical problem, shouldn't we want to confront it? Not necessarily, because confronting medical conditions is difficult. Nevertheless, the first step in preventing more serious complications down the road is to reach the stage where we accept that *acting now* could save our lives.

We understand enough about the risk factors for CKD that we know some things we can do to significantly reduce the chances of CKD *before it occurs*. Being educated about health risks is a good start (chapter 3). In this chapter, I outline some specific ways to address these risks. Sound medical practices may reduce the risk of CKD and address many other health issues, such as the harmful consequences of diabetes, hypertension, and heart disease. In addition to safeguarding your health, you need to have regular medical checkups and treat any underlying causes of CKD, especially if you have a family history of CKD, diabetes, or hypertension or are a member of an at-risk population.

Weight Loss, Diet, and Exercise

Hypertension is one of the main contributors to CKD, no matter what the primary cause of the loss of kidney function. Although factors related to diabetes, glomerular diseases, and PKD can destroy kidney function, hypertension can accelerate the decline. A major contributor to hypertension is obesity (chapter 3).

Obesity can increase blood pressure in several ways. For one, the heart must work harder to move blood through a large body. In addition, the renin-angiotensin and adrenaline systems become overactive (chapter 2). In people with diabetes, insulin resistance is a factor. Fat deposits can apply pressure on the outside walls of blood vessels, increasing resistance to blood flow. Finally, increased salt consumption accompanies overeating; excess salt intake promotes water retention, further contributing to hypertension. The bottom line? Overweight people at risk of CKD must lose weight.

Granted, losing weight is easier said than done. Books and magazines tout various ways to shed unwanted pounds, and I am not going to evaluate their claims here. I will confirm, however, the mantra of every weight-reducing diet: *to lose weight, you must burn more calories than you consume.* This used to mean adopting a healthy, low-calorie, low-fat diet and an exercise program. However, in the last decade, a shift from low-fat to low-carbohydrate diets (low-carb) has become more accepted. Moreover, a carbohydrate-rich diet can worsen CKD, especially in the late stages.[1]

People on low-carb diets lose more weight than those on low-fat diets.[2] The rationale for a low-carb diet is that fats cannot be made in the body without carbohydrates, so reducing them in the diet would logically lower the amount of fats made by the body. That does not mean that you can eat all the fat you want. Remember, you still have to burn more calories than you consume. However, some fats, so called healthy fats, are needed for a balanced diet, especially those from fish, olive oil, and nuts, such as walnuts and pecans. No-carb diets can be dangerous, too, if you are on them for too long.

The real culprit in dieting and maintaining good health is sugar. It can come from a variety of sources, such as sucrose and high-fructose corn syrup found in sweetened beverages, cereal, fruit juices, desserts, and sugar added at the table. Added sugars in foods are overconsumed by the public and contribute to many health conditions, such as diabetes and obesity. According to the World Health Organization (WHO), malnutrition is caused in part by consuming a high proportion of the diet as sugar-enriched foods rather than a more balanced diet, especially in low- to middle-income countries.[3] The WHO has recommended that adults and children keep sugar content to about 5 percent of their diets or about 32 g/day (grams per day) for adults and 19–24 g/day for children, aged 4–11. For perspective, a 20-ounce bottle of Coca-Cola has 65 g of sugar! In the United States, sugar consumption is 114 g/day for those without CKD and about 100 g/day for those with CKD from all causes and for those at middle stages of CKD.[4] That is more than three times the recommended amounts! Fortunately, to help you trim unwanted calories from added sugars, the US Food and Drug Administration (FDA) has released a new food label (figure 5.1) that will be discussed in a later section of this chapter.

One final note on dieting: Don't be fooled into thinking that using noncaloric artificial sweeteners will get around the problems with sugar. On the one hand, our brains are not easily tricked into responding to a sweet-tasting, artificial sweetener, especially when we are hungry. What can happen later is an overconsumption of sugar, because the body did not get the calories it needed.[5] On the other hand, artificial sweeteners can have their own potentially harmful effects on the body. Ever since cyclamates were banned in 1969 because of their cancer risk, concern has continued about the safety of artificial sweeteners. Aspartame (NutraSweet), approved by the FDA in 1974, has some common side effects, such as headaches and gastrointestinal problems. In addition, aspartame can accelerate a decline in kidney function in older women.[6] Whether these findings apply to the general population awaits further research. Other artificial sweeteners, such as sucralose (Splenda) and Stevia have been certified safe by the FDA. Some people, especially those who have or are at risk of diabetes, may be better off just drinking water and allowing the body to get used to lowering sugar intake.

The other key component for losing weight and maintaining good health is exercise. We have all heard about the benefits of exercise, such as losing weight, lowering blood pressure, increasing endurance, enhancing physical strength, and improving heart function and bone density.

What kind of exercise is best? Some exercise is better than no exercise. In general, the National Kidney Foundation, recommends exercising 30–60 minutes on most days of the week. Even walking is beneficial. For those who are capable, more intense training can be useful. However, weight loss is modest without intensive, calorie-burning exercise.[7] To put this concept in a real-world situation, if you have ever been on a treadmill that counts calories, you have probably noticed you had to walk or run for quite a while to burn 100–200 calories. Compare that to a candy bar with 200–300 calories, and it is easy to see the limits of exercise in weight loss. In fact, cutting calories in your diet will do more for weight loss than exercise will, unless the exercise is done at intense levels. Nevertheless, the other health benefits from exercise are worth the effort.

Can you exercise if you have CKD? The answer is usually yes, depending on your physical status. Accumulating evidence suggests that regular exercise may reduce the risk of the following: death from all causes, rapid decline in kidney function in non-dialysis patients, frailty and muscle loss, and loss of transplanted kidneys.[8] Even walking can have similar effects.[9] In addition, exercise improves cardiovascular function in those with advanced CKD.[10] Cardiovascular disease is the most common cause of death in CKD. So, exercise is well worth the effort for CKD patients.

To finish this discussion of obesity and weight loss, I have my own story. I was once obese. In my thirties and early forties, I became too fond of junk food. Over time, I gained 60 to 70 pounds above my ideal weight. I had a poor self-image and had high blood pressure, but what got my attention was an incident one evening as I climbed a flight of stairs to bed. I felt so winded that I could barely breathe. I realized then that if I didn't do something about my weight, I might not make it to my sixties.

In consultation with my physician, I changed my diet and started exercising. Changing my diet took time. My body had become accustomed to all the sugar and fat that I had been eating. Eventually, my new diet stuck, and I reached a point where eating junk food made me sick. Sticking to my diet didn't mean I had to deprive myself of anything. When I had a craving for a certain food, I would eat it but only very small portions. Allowing myself this luxury helped me avoid consuming extra calories.

Beginning an exercise regimen was also a challenge, largely because I didn't know how to do it effectively. So, I hired a personal trainer who accepted no excuses from me about not coming to the gym as scheduled. The first few months were very frustrating. I didn't lose any weight at all for three months, even though I ate a low-calorie diet and vigorously exercised. It took that long to trick my body into accepting my lower caloric intake instead of my usual high caloric consumption. After that, I lost 30 pounds in the next few months. Eventually, I lost the extra pounds and returned to a normal weight. I am now in my seventies, sixteen years post-transplant. I've kept the weight off with a healthy, low-carb diet, although when I have a craving for something sweet, I eat only a small portion size. I continue to exercise regularly. I do CrossFit, but that can be difficult to sustain, especially as you get older or you have health problems such as CKD. I admit it: exercise can be very difficult to start and maintain, but it is worth the effort. Exercise helped me feel stronger, which helped me deal with all the problems of CKD.

In summary, I know firsthand how difficult it is to lose weight. There are no quick tricks, either. To lose weight and keep it off requires a permanent change in lifestyle, involving diet and exercise. You must make losing weight a priority and you must be motivated, disciplined, and determined to get to a healthy weight. With the help of your doctor, a nutritionist, perhaps a personal trainer, and the support of friends and family, you, too, can lose weight. It takes a long-term commitment and patience.

Sodium, Protein, and Phosphorus Restriction

Reducing your intake of specific foods may help you lose weight and may also reduce the strain on your kidneys and prolong their function.

The first dietary change that people with kidney disease should make is to restrict sodium intake. Regardless of the source of the sodium, whether it's from table salt, sea salt, Himalayan salt, or any other exotic salts, it is the same substance. Although the specialty salts are processed differently and may have some beneficial minerals, the products still have the same amount of sodium.

The American Heart Association recommends that we eat less than 1,500 mg (milligrams) of sodium a day, whereas the WHO recommends less than 2,000 mg a day. The WHO also recommends that children consume proportionally less sodium, based on their size and activity. Global consumption of sodium averages more than twice the recommended levels, with the highest intake in the Republic of Georgia and the lowest in Kenya.[11] Americans ingest more than 3,400 mg of sodium a day. This overconsumption of sodium has contributed to high blood pressure and heart disease and in turn to CKD. Moreover, restricting sodium can reduce blood pressure, protein in the urine, and the decline in kidney function in CKD.[12]

The WHO also recommends ingesting at least 3,500 mg of potassium a day, because it helps to eliminate sodium. That goal may be difficult to meet, however, even with eating a lot of high potassium foods, such as bananas, potatoes, oranges and orange juice, and dairy products.[13] Moreover, as CKD progresses, potassium intake may have to be reduced (chapter 4), so guidance from your nephrologist is needed.

The biggest problem in reducing sodium intake is that so much of what we buy and eat is loaded with it, so it can be difficult to avoid. In addition, eating less sodium can be hard to get used to. Like eating fewer calories, you can condition yourself to prefer the taste of foods with less sodium. The biggest culprits providing excess sodium are meals in restaurants and processed or prepared foods.

Restaurants often serve extremely large portions of food, and their meals are also often excessively salty. While you don't need to avoid eating in restaurants, there are ways you can minimize your caloric and sodium intake. First, if your meal is too large, divide it in half or in thirds and take the rest home for subsequent meals. Avoid ordering menu items that come with sauces, which are often full of fat and sodium. You may also ask the chef to avoid salting your food as much as possible. (You can always add some salt to taste if the food is too bland.) Eat grilled or broiled food instead of fried food, which is generally high in fat. (If the grilled or broiled food is coated with fat and salt as in many marinades, however, it may still be unhealthy.) Finally, experiment with healthy cuisines that you may not normally eat. You may discover foods that you really like and that are more nutritious and less salty than your normal fare. On the bright side, some restaurant chains have been posting nutritional information on their menus. This is a step forward and can help you reduce sodium intake when you eat their meal items.

Processed foods often have too much sodium. This is especially true of frozen meals and canned foods and soups. You don't need to avoid these convenience foods completely but learn how to read the nutrition labels. If you normally eat three meals a day, remember that a single meal cannot contain more than 500–600 mg of sodium and still remain within the daily guideline. Of course, if you eat more than three meals a day—a practice that is often recommended in dieting—each small meal must have proportionally less sodium. Several companies, such as Healthy Choice and Lean Cuisine, sell frozen meals with lower sodium content than other companies' products. Read and compare labels. Canned foods often have a lot of sodium, but you can significantly reduce the sodium by discarding any liquid in the cans and then by rinsing the contents. Obviously, this approach will not work with canned soups, which generally should be avoided. If you like soup, make your own with fresh ingredients and as little salt as possible.

Governments have become involved in trying to reduce sodium consumption in their populations. The FDA has proposed a voluntary reduction of sodium in food products. This approach has worked in other countries, such as Great Britain and Finland. The results have been promising, with a significant reduction in blood pressure and heart disease in those countries,[14] but more time is needed to determine whether the programs are really working in the long term. In the meantime, continue to read the food labels to find the best products for you.

Finally, some recent developments suggest that other means of controlling sodium intake are possible. For example, researchers have tested monitors that can measure sodium in food[15] and drugs that can block the absorption of sodium.[16] When dietary restriction and diuretics are insufficient to keep sodium overload low, these approaches may hold some promise in the future and may postpone the start of dialysis or transplantation in some people.

Reducing protein in the diet may also be helpful in postponing the progression of CKD.[17] Because kidneys normally filter protein and return it to the blood, lower levels of protein may reduce the workload on your kidneys. People with diabetes or glomerular diseases (where protein spills into the urine, reflecting kidney damage) can improve their health by eating less protein. In addition, you might eat soy or other plant protein, such as legumes and whole grains, rather than animal protein. For the most part, reducing the amount of protein you consume has little downside risk and might be beneficial to your health. However, people with advanced kidney failure should be cautious. Reducing your protein intake may result in insufficient caloric intake and may put you at significant risk of malnutrition.[18] In addition, the value of protein restriction may depend on the cause of the CKD. Talk to your nephrologist and your dietitian to strike the right balance.

As we learned in chapter 2, phosphorus in the form of phosphate is an important element in many energy-producing reactions of the body. Because we consume more phosphorus than we need, the kidney must excrete the excess amount. As a result, high blood phosphorus levels are a warning sign for CKD. Limiting phosphorus intake can help take the load off your kidneys. When a person's kidney function is poor or the person is on dialysis (chapter 6), it is even more important to limit phosphorus consumption, since high phosphorus raises the risk of death.[19] Cola drinks and dairy products are a main source of phosphorus and may have to be consumed in small amounts only. Rice milk and almond milk are suitable substitutes for skim milk, whereas soy milk contains too much phosphorus.

Finally, a question often asked by those with CKD is whether they should drink alcoholic beverages. The answer is *maybe*, depending on the underlying disease and stage of CKD. According to the National Kidney Foundation, drinking alcohol in high amounts can raise blood pressure, dry out the body, and lead to liver damage. Usually, drinking no more than two drinks per day for men and one drink per day for women and those over age 65 will not cause problems. When drinking three or more drinks per day, considered heavy drinking, or when binge drinking four to five drinks within two hours, the risk for kidney damage and/or CKD increases. Moreover, those on certain medications or with liver disease are advised not to drink alcohol at all. Check with your doctor for what course is best for you.

Reading Food Labels

It's easy to eat the wrong foods, in part because we do not under-stand what's in the food we're eating. Learning to read a food label is one way to help avoid eating harmful foods. Figure 5.1 shows an example of the new food label, which was required for most packaging by the beginning of 2020. The figure compares this new label with the one that has been around for years. Several items and changes on the label are particularly pertinent for people with failing kidneys as well as for people trying to lose weight.

First, check the serving size. It can be easy to buy an item that looks as if it is a single serving when it is not. A small package of snacks or bottle of soda often represents more than one serving. In the case of two servings, eating the entire item means consuming two servings and double the calories, carbs, fat, and salt of the single serving as gauged by the food manufacturer.

If you are trying to lose weight or prevent type 2 diabetes, note that the food label now lists the amount of added sugar. This is a huge change and a positive step for helping people improve their health. Many foods have their own natural sugar content, but producers often add sugar to make them sweeter, especially if the product is diluted with water, such as many fruit juices and of course sugary sodas. Often, juices have very little fruit in them. Try to avoid consuming items with added sugar. They have little or no nutritional value.

Another major and valuable change for those with CKD is a new listing for potassium. Previously, some manufacturers volun-tarily listed potassium content, but now it is required for all foods. You can now apportion the right amount of potassium into your diet, based on recommendations from your doctor and nutritionist.

Unfortunately, food manufacturers are still not required to list the phosphorus content per serving on their food labels. This poses a unique challenge for people with CKD and in the clinical management of the disease. Serum phosphate is a measure of the

FIGURE 5.1. The New Food Label: Old Label (*left*), New Label (*right*)

Nutrition Facts	
Serving Size 2/3 cup (55g)	
Servings Per Container About 8	
Amount Per serving	
Calories 230	Calories from Fat 72
	% Daily Value*
Total Fat 8g	**12%**
Saturated Fat 1g	**5%**
Trans Fat 0g	
Cholesterol 0mg	**0%**
Sodium 160mg	**7%**
Total Carbohydrate 37g	**12%**
Dietary Fiber 4g	**16%**
Sugars 1g	
Protein 3g	
Vitamin A	10%
Vitamin C	8%
Calcium	20%
Iron	45%

* Percent Daily Values are based on a 2,000 calorie diet. Your daily value may be higher or lower depending on your calorie needs.

	Calories:	2,000	2,500
Total Fat	Less than	65g	80g
Sat Fat	Less than	20g	25g
Cholesterol	Less than	300mg	300mg
Sodium	Less than	2,400mg	2,400mg
Total Carbohydrate		300g	375g
Dietary Fiber		25g	30g

Nutrition Facts	
8 servings per container	
Serving size **2/3 cup (55g)**	
Amount per serving	
Calories	**230**
	% Daily Value*
Total Fat 8g	**10%**
Saturated Fat 1g	**5%**
Trans Fat 0g	
Cholesterol 0g	**0%**
Sodium 160g	**7%**
Total Carbohydrate 37g	**13%**
Dietary Fiber 4g	**14%**
Total Sugars 12g	
Includes 10g Added Sugars	**20%**
Protein 3g	
Vitamin D 2mcg	10%
Calcium 260mg	20%
Iron 8mg	45%
Potassium 235mg	6%

* The % Daily Value (DV) tells you how much a nutrient in a serving of food contributes to a daily diet. 2,000 calories a day is used for general nutrition advice.

adequacy of treatment.[20] A simple change in the food label to include phosphorus content would be helpful. Some manufacturers list it voluntarily, helping you to know which products are safe to eat and which items to avoid. Hopefully, the FDA will plan to include phosphorus in any future food labels. To help you make better choices, some foods high and low in potassium and phosphorus are found in tables 6.1 to 6.4.

Fat, cholesterol, and sodium content on food packaging have not changed with the new label. These nutrients should be consumed only in small amounts if you have CKD. *Trans* fats should be avoided completely. A high-fat and high-salt diet can lead to the formation of fat deposits in blood vessels and to high blood pressure, heart disease, and some cancers. Some fats, however—those designated as monounsaturated or polyunsaturated such as olive oil—may be beneficial.

The listing of vitamins has changed. Instead of listing vitamins A and C, they have been replaced by vitamin D. This change is useful to people with CKD. Adding the amounts of vitamin D, calcium, iron, and potassium to the label allows you to plan better choices during the day. Some people do not get enough vitamins and minerals in their diets and may need to take supplements to satisfy their daily requirements.

Finally, the footnote at the bottom of the old food label has been deleted. This is too bad because it provided basic nutritional information, based on the advice of experts, on the upper and lower limits you should consume daily, depending on the number of calories consumed. These values provided comparisons among food items, so it was easier to identify which foods were best for your diet. Hopefully, the FDA will reconsider removing this information.

Treating the Underlying Causes of Chronic Kidney Disease

Preventing CKD depends on effectively treating its underlying causes. There are many ways to treat hypertension in a person who has no other underlying diseases. However, there are not as many ways to treat diabetes, glomerular diseases, and PKD. Clinical researchers are always working to develop new, more effective drugs. They do this by first studying relevant mechanisms in animal trials. If the results are promising, they move ahead to clinical trials using human volunteers. The federal government has established a website that lists current clinical trials (www.clinicaltrials.gov). On this website, you can find information about current research and applications. There are some promising new approaches to treating the underlying diseases that can lead to CKD. The sections that follow address specific diseases, examples of long-standing treatments, new drugs introduced in the past decade, and medications or devices currently in development. This discussion is not meant to be all inclusive but to provide a flavor of what is available or under development. As you read these descriptions, remember that, in scientific and medical research, new treatment possibilities emerge while others become dead ends. With all the treatment options described in this chapter, consult your health care team to determine whether you are a candidate for any of them.

Diabetes

The first line of treatment for diabetes is controlling glucose and insulin levels. For people with mild diabetes, a healthy diet is the first step, especially eating a low-carb diet.[21] The body's supply of glucose and insulin is further regulated through medications that are taken orally. None of these treatments is a cure for diabetes, however. Clinical trials are under way to find better treatments or a cure for both type 1 and type 2 diabetes.

Type 1 Diabetes. The standard approach to treating type 1 diabetes is managing blood glucose levels within a narrow range and minimizing damage to the insulin-producing beta cells in the pancreas that the body's own immune system is destroying (chapter 3). In the past, glucose monitoring during the day with frequent blood checks and injections of insulin could be difficult and sometimes led to glucose levels that were either too high or too low. Considerable progress has been made to reduce this problem by employing insulin pumps, new forms of insulin that adjust blood glucose levels at different speeds, new medications, and pancreatic islet transplantation. I will briefly discuss these options in turn.

Insulin can be administered in several ways. In addition to injection with a standard needle, insulin can be administered with a device like a spring-loaded pen, an inhaler, or an infusion pump attached to a tube and a needle inserted under the skin. Some of these pumps have become quite sophisticated. Known as an artificial pancreas, they control blood glucose using sensors to monitor the concentration of glucose, and the pump automatically injects insulin when glucose levels get too high. In some cases, glucagon, a hormone that stimulates the conversion of glycogen to glucose in the liver, can be included to raise glucose in the blood when levels are too low. This new approach is effective in providing good glucose control over a twenty-four-hour period.[22]

Different forms of insulin, called insulin analogs, have been developed that have different characteristics from natural insulin.[23] Depending on how active a person is, the analog to use can be short or long acting. The short-acting ones can be used around meals to prevent glucose spiking, whereas the long-acting ones can be used at bedtime. Some new analogs are being developed in experimental animals that are "smart" forms of insulin. Researchers have created insulin molecules that work only when glucose levels are high[24] or restrict glucose uptake into cells once levels are in the normal range.[25] This path could be a powerful new direction for research in maintaining normal glucose levels.

Finding a treatment beyond insulin to treat type 1 diabetes has been elusive. Part of the problem is determining the best time to intervene; for example, when evidence is found for potential disease development, at early stages after diagnosis, or during later stages when damage to the pancreas has already been established. Another problem is not knowing all the mechanisms involved in the development of type 1 diabetes. Although a host of different treatment approaches have been tried over the past decade, the results have been mixed.[26]

Clinical trials on type 1 diabetes are testing better treatment options to protect the insulin-producing beta cells from being destroyed by the body's own antibodies. The current treatment approach of suppressing the immune system interferes with all immune reactions and makes people more vulnerable to infections. The goal of the latest research is to block specific pathways in the immune response that attack beta cells rather than suppress the entire immune system. Research is slowly identifying which pathways might be the best targets for therapeutic intervention as well as for effective new medications. Another way to treat type 1 diabetes is to desensitize the specific immune response that damages beta cells so that the pathway is less responsive to autoimmune attack. Desensitizing the immune response also reduces the chance that a transplanted organ will be rejected by the body (chapter 7). So far, clinical trials have either yielded disappointing results or are still in early stages, so results are not yet available.

Another approach for treating type 1 diabetes is testing drugs used successfully for treating type 2 diabetes. These drugs will be discussed later in this section, and their potential looks encouraging.

Finally, the use of pancreatic islet cell transplants for treating type 1 diabetes has shown considerable progress over the past decade.[27] With islet transplants, islet cells from deceased donors are infused into a recipient to restore normal insulin secretion. The recipient has to take steroids to suppress system-wide immune responses to these "foreign" islet cells. Clinical research has shown that islet cell transplants are effective in 50 to 70 percent of cases, and even after five years, patients no longer need insulin. Islet transplants are intended mostly for those with poor control of glucose levels, severe episodes of low blood sugar, and a lack of awareness of these episodes. Eventually, islet transplants may provide a potential cure for type 1 diabetes.

In the future, it may be possible to take human skin cells from a person with type 1 diabetes and convert them into pancreatic beta cells for transplant back into that person.[28] In mice, these newly made beta cells produced insulin, which was released in response to glucose and protected the animals from developing diabetes in an experimental model. If this approach becomes feasible in humans, it would be possible to cure type 1 diabetes using your own skin cells that have been converted to insulin-producing cells. Since the skin cells come from you, then the beta cells would not be recognized by your immune system as "foreign," so there would be no need for antirejection medications.

Type 2 Diabetes. Researchers are working to develop better drugs that can control cellular responsiveness to insulin. People with type 2 diabetes are insulin resistant and may benefit from oral medications that improve insulin responsiveness. Insulin responsiveness is a prime target for research to help with type 2 diabetes. Although these types of drugs, such as metformin, have been available for decades, they have not been very effective in people with severe diabetes. For these people, insulin injections are needed to control blood glucose levels. But there is good news.

New classes of drugs have been developed that not only control blood sugar but also reduce cardiovascular risk and stabilize the progression of CKD.[29] From a kidney-protective perspective, the most exciting new drugs are the so-called SGLT2 (sodium glucose cotransporter 2) inhibitors, such as empagliflozin (Jardiance), canagliflozin (Invokana), and dapagliflozin (Farxiga). These drugs work on the kidney by enhancing the removal of glucose from the body, thereby reducing high blood glucose and high kidney glucose levels. In addition, they reduce the risk of CKD and retard the progression of CKD caused by diabetes and by other kidney diseases.[30] As new drugs, their long-term effects on the body have not been determined. Thus, they can be used only in CKD stages G1 through G3a (table 4.2). They might also have the added benefits of enhancing weight loss and lowering blood pressure. Other new drugs, which work through different mechanisms, are also available for treatment of diabetes, although some of these drugs should not be used if you have CKD. Management of type 2 diabetes can be a complicated process, so your doctor can help you determine whether these new drugs are appropriate for you, especially if you have CKD or are at risk of developing CKD.

As drugs that are more effective in controlling insulin resistance are approved, more people with diabetes might be able to eliminate or postpone the need to take insulin. In the long term, these drugs may prevent CKD entirely in those with diabetes.

Another interesting development in treating type 2 diabetes is bariatric surgery, especially for those who are very obese and/or whose diabetes is severe.[31] Bariatric surgery, also called gastric bypass surgery, can be performed several different ways, but the common feature is reducing the size of the stomach. It has been shown to effectively induce weight loss by restricting caloric intake. In addition, bariatric surgery can be effective in treating type 2 diabetes, lowering blood pressure and blood fats, and reducing cardiovascular problems. Initially, bariatric surgery looked like a cure for type 2 diabetes, but over time, many patients began having high blood glucose levels again. Even then, though, their diabetes was less severe. These findings do not mean that eligible people should not consider bariatric surgery. The National Institutes of Health recommends that those with a body mass index (chapter 3) of 30–35 with accompanied diabetes should consider this surgery. With any surgery though, there are risks, so if you are considering bariatric surgery, discuss all aspects of the program, which may include glucose-lowering agents, with your health care team.

Another consideration when treating type 2 diabetes is whether obesity should be treated before diabetes and other medical consequences. According to new guidelines developed by the American Association of Clinical Endocrinologists and the American College of Endocrinology, obesity should be treated first before other obesity-related problems.[32] The reason behind this recommendation is that by successfully treating obesity, the other medical issues might either resolve themselves or be lessened in severity. Given the complexity of this issue, diabetes management should continue until enough weight loss is attained. Again, consult with your health care team to develop the best treatment plan.

High Blood Pressure

The usual treatment for high blood pressure starts with diet, especially a low-salt diet and especially for those who are obese. Although obesity can contribute to hypertension, not everyone with hypertension is overweight. In obese people and in people with hypertension, however, diet alone may not lower blood pressure to the recommended level. Some people, therefore, must take medications to control high blood pressure.

As discussed in chapter 3, the guidelines for treating high blood pressure have been controversial. As a result, deciding when to begin treatment should be done in close consultation with your doctor, weighing the benefits of treatment against the pitfalls and side effects of medications. Luckily, the treatment of high blood pressure has evolved over the past four decades, and today there are many classes of medications working through different mechanisms to control blood pressure. Although a single medication may be effective in controlling high blood pressure, clinical research has shown that a combination of medications may be needed to produce the desired outcome. Some classes of medications may be better than others in protecting kidney function. However, the use of a diuretic (water pills), such as hydrochlorothiazide (Microzide) is often the initial treatment to help reduce both fluid retention in the body and blood pressure.

As discussed in chapter 2, a biochemical process initially mediated by the kidney can cause hypertension. This process involves the release of the hormone renin from the kidney. Renin activates angiotensin synthetic pathways, whereby angiotensin II constricts blood vessels and increases blood pressure.

The two ways to interfere with the ability of angiotensin II to elevate blood pressure are (1) to block the production of angiotensin II or (2) to reduce the action of angiotensin II on blood vessels. Medications that block the formation of angiotensin II are called *angiotensin-converting enzyme*, or *ACE inhibitors*. One such medication is lisinopril (Zestril and Prinivil). These drugs have been in use for many years, have been well studied, and might be especially beneficial in protecting kidney function. Another drug that blocks angiotensin II receptors is losartan (Cozaar). This drug also reduces blood pressure effectively. Using both drugs together, however, does not provide improved treatment and is not recommended.

The other drug classes that can reduce blood pressure do so by relaxing blood vessels directly or by altering heart rate and the amount of blood the heart ejects with each beat (cardiac output)—or through a combination of these effects. At the cellular level, all of these drugs work by blocking receptors that normally translate the signals of the body's hormones or chemical transmitters into a physiological response. Two classes of drugs that lower blood pressure act on the heart and, to some extent, on the blood vessels directly. One class, named beta-blockers, slows the heart rate and reduces cardiac output, thereby lessening the burden on the heart and reducing blood pressure. Metoprolol (Lopressor) and carvedilol (Coreg) are commonly prescribed beta-blockers. The other class of drugs acting on the heart and blood vessels includes the calcium-channel blockers, such as amlodipine (Norvasc). These drugs prevent the inflow of calcium into cells that stimulate the contraction of muscle in the heart and blood vessels, thereby lowering blood pressure.

As we learned earlier, hypertension is often difficult to treat with only one class of drug. To control your hypertension, you may need to take several different classes of drugs with different actions and possibly others as well, including, alpha-blockers such as terazosin (Hytrin), which acts directly on the blood vessels; others, which work through the brain; and minoxidil (Loniten), which directly opens blood vessels. Your doctor may use trial and error to determine the best treatment for your hypertension.

Sometimes, high blood pressure can be resistant to medications (systolic blood pressure greater than 160 after using three medications). An interesting new development for this problem is renal sympathetic denervation.[33] This procedure cuts the nerve to the renal artery and removes nerve impulses to the kidney, thereby removing a stimulus involved in raising systolic blood pressure. Although this treatment has been controversial, it may someday be an alternative or a supplement to medications to treat resistant high blood pressure.

Glomerular Diseases

New treatments for glomerular diseases are emerging, too. The approach of these treatments varies depending on the original source of the disease (chapter 3). Glomerular diseases are inflammatory diseases that lead to scarring of the glomerulus, and most of the treatment options use steroids to reduce inflammation. Most clinical trials on inflammation focus on inflammatory diseases such as lupus. Here, like the studies of type 1 diabetes, researchers are examining pathways within the immune system to find the most selective approach to minimize or slow the scarring without using steroids.

Current treatment of glomerular diseases first involves treating any identified, underlying cause. Often, treatments include reducing high blood pressure with ACE inhibitors, controlling blood sugar, and using low-protein diets to reduce protein loss through the kidneys.

Recent exciting findings from clinical trials suggest that two new drugs provide a better treatment for lupus nephritis than current treatment alone. In late-stage clinical trials, both belimumab and voclosporin show promising results in reducing the decline in kidney function.[34] Hopefully, these current clinical trials will provide better specific options for treatment in the future.

Polycystic Kidney Disease

Clinical trials to find medications to retard cyst growth in PKD patients are pursuing what is perhaps the most promising approach for treating a major cause of kidney failure. Having developed a better understanding of the underlying mechanisms of how cysts form in the kidneys, researchers have been looking for ways to shrink the size of the cysts.

The most important advance in the treatment of PKD is the newly FDA-approved drug tolvaptan (Jynarque). Tolvaptan works by blocking the action of the hormone *vasopressin*.[35] Vasopressin, which is released from the pituitary gland to conserve fluid in the body, does so by stimulating cellular mechanisms that can cause cyst formation and growth in people with mutations in their PKD genes (chapter 3). Indeed, vasopressin levels are higher in PKD patients. Since tolvaptan promotes urination, clinical trials are ongoing to see whether high water intake can produce the same effect as tolvaptan. Stay tuned. Tolvaptan use is not for everyone, so discuss with your nephrologist to see if you are a candidate.

NEW RESEARCH ON THE underlying causes of CKD and the continued development of potential treatments offer hope to people in fear of losing their kidney function and of facing dialysis or transplantation. Someday, we hope, there will be no need for dialysis clinics and transplant lists and less need for expensive and invasive medical interventions. In the future, the lives of many people with kidney diseases will improve.

In the meantime, people approaching kidney failure must examine the choices available to replace their impending kidney failure. Chapters 6 and 7 cover what you can expect with dialysis and transplantation and introduce helpful coping skills.

CHAPTER 6

Dialysis

U NTIL RECENT DECADES, few seriously ill people got a second chance at life. It wasn't until the twentieth century that effective treatments were developed for many diseases. Now, antibiotics and other medical interventions routinely preserve life for many who might otherwise die. Like people with serious infections and people with cancer, people with chronic kidney disease (CKD) are now having much longer life expectancies than they would have had in the past. Then, the kidneys of people with CKD deteriorated to the point called kidney failure when *uremia*, an excessive buildup of toxins in the blood, resulted in death.

Today, however, there are treatments for kidney failure, including dialysis and transplantation. Although tested as early as the nineteenth century, dialyzing blood to reduce uremia only became a useful treatment for kidney failure in the 1960s. Now dialysis is in use all over the United States and is available to anyone who needs it. According to the latest statistics from the National Institutes of Health, over 554,000 people were on some form of dialysis at the end of 2019.[1]

There are two forms of dialysis to treat kidney failure: peritoneal dialysis and hemodialysis. Both forms of dialysis move toxins across a barrier through which only some substances can pass. The following section explains the basic concepts of dialysis.

How Dialysis Works

Dialysis involves filtration. Start with a basic concept: imagine a tank of water into which you carefully place a drop of ink in one corner of the tank. The concentrated ink tends to diffuse over time throughout the entire container of water until it reaches the same concentration in all parts of the tank (figure 6.1, *top*).

Now insert a barrier, through which nothing can pass, in the middle of the tank. The ink diffuses throughout only half the container, as shown in figure 6.1 (*bottom*). If, however, you punch tiny holes into the barrier, ink will flow through them—if the ink molecules are smaller than the holes. If the molecules are smaller, they disperse throughout the entire container of water (as in figure 6.1, *top*). If the holes are too small for the ink molecules to pass through, the ink remains on one side of the barrier (figure 6.1, *bottom*).

Increasing the volume of the left side of the tank causes the ink to diffuse faster through the barrier until the *concentration* of ink is equal on both sides, while the *amount* of ink is reduced on the right side (figure 6.2). For example, if you place 3 grams of ink in the right side of the tank with 1 L (liter) of water and the ink moves through the barrier to the other side with 2 L of water, the concentration of ink will eventually be equal on both sides of the barrier. This means only 1 gram remains on the original side of the barrier, and the remaining 2 grams have crossed the barrier. Thus, on the original side, the concentration of ink declined from 3 g/L to 1 g/L, while on the other side the concentration rose from 0 g/2 L to 2 g/2 L, or 1 g/L. (The *amount* of ink on each side of the barrier rather than the *concentration* of ink is shown in figure 6.2. Because the concentration would be equal on each side, if concentrations were illustrated, both sides would be the same shade, as in the top part of figure 6.1.)

This concept, called *dialysis*, has been used for years by biochemists to purify chemicals. Like the ink analogy, *dialysis* involves a semipermeable membrane (a barrier with holes) that allows some substances to pass through and not others, depending on the size of the molecules involved. To accomplish this, the chemical needing purification is placed into a small sac made of the membranous material (the barrier from above) through which the substance to be purified cannot pass. Next, the sac is placed in a volume of appropriate solution much larger than the volume of solution in the sac. The impurities that can pass through the membrane will flow until the concentration is equal on both sides of the membrane but reducing their *amount* inside the sac. For maximum efficiency, the solution is changed frequently to allow for the greatest removal of

FIGURE 6.1. Dialysis as Filtration I. With no barriers, a substance will diffuse uniformly (*top*). If a barrier is added, diffusion will only occur in half the container (*bottom*).

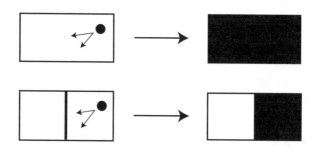

FIGURE 6.2. Dialysis as Filtration II. This figure shows the *amount* of ink on each side of the barrier rather than the *concentration* of ink. Since the concentration would be equal on each side, if concentrations (rather than amounts) of ink were illustrated, both sides would be the same color, as in the top part of figure 6.1.

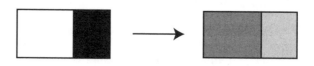

the contaminants in the sac. When the exchanges are successively repeated, nearly all the impurities eventually will be removed.

This is the same basic approach to filtering the blood of people with kidney failure. Early studies in the 1940s, using this principle of dialysis to clean human blood, used pig intestines as the semipermeable membrane, with the blood passing through the interior part. The intestines were placed in big wooden vats of solution composed of salts and buffers compatible with blood. Other laboratories tried using cellophane. The idea was to remove the toxins without removing cells and important proteins from the blood. This approach proved more difficult than simple biochemical dialysis, but over time, with further refinements and miniaturizing the process, the modern forms of dialysis were born.

Today, the most common forms of dialysis are peritoneal dialysis and hemodialysis. Hemodialysis is more routinely used than peritoneal dialysis. In 2019, 89.4 percent of those being treated for kidney failure in the United States were on hemodialysis and 10.6 percent were on peritoneal dialysis.[1] Not all countries have dialysis readily available to those with kidney failure. Restrictions are based on the lack of funds, especially in low-income countries, to pay for dialysis.[2] Emphasis in these countries is on reducing the progression of CKD.[3] Often, those needing dialysis are encouraged to start with peritoneal dialysis or the increasingly used home hemodialysis, because they are less expensive than in-center hemodialysis. In the United States, home hemodialysis has been slowly adopted, accounting for only about 8 percent of patients with kidney failure.

Peritoneal Dialysis

The principles of peritoneal dialysis are the same as described earlier, but the application is a bit more complicated. Like the biochemical approach to dialysis, *peritoneal dialysis* takes advantage of the semipermeable membrane that lines the peritoneal cavity of the abdomen. Some substances can pass through it, others cannot. Tiny blood vessels are embedded in this peritoneal membrane. The blood from the body is analogous to the contents of the membranous sac described previously. A solution, called the *dialysate*, is placed in the abdomen, allowing the toxins in the blood to flow through the peritoneal membrane into the solution (figure 6.3). This occurs because the concentration of toxins in the blood is higher than it is in the dialysate (as in figure 6.2). To avoid loss of needed substances in the blood, the dialysate contains salts and buffers in concentrations equivalent to those normally found in the blood, creating equal concentrations of these substances on both sides of the membrane.

Because fluid balance is compromised in people with kidney failure, dialysis must also remove excess water from the body. In peritoneal dialysis, the dialysate contains glucose (sugar) to help remove the excess water. Because the concentration of glucose exceeds the concentration in the blood, some glucose passes into the body. However, excess fluid in the blood flows through the peritoneal membrane into the dialysate to dilute the glucose until glucose concentrations stabilize on each side of the membrane. To remove more fluid, higher concentrations of glucose are needed. The rate of diffusion of toxins into the dialysate declines with time, so the dialysate must be exchanged up to five times a day to maximize the removal of the toxins.

Before peritoneal dialysis can be performed, a surgeon or interventional radiologist (if the patient has had no previous surgeries) must place a special *catheter* inside the abdominal wall (figure 6.4). The catheter is generally placed in the lower abdomen. The part of the catheter inside the abdominal wall is either straight or curled like a pig's tail and has holes in it, whereas on the outside the catheter is straight, solid, and flexible and has a hole only at the outside tip. The hole in the abdomen through which the catheter exits is known as the *exit site*. The subcutaneous (below the skin) and peritoneal cuffs are sewn into the abdominal wall, thus holding

FIGURE 6.3. Dialysate Flowing into the Abdomen

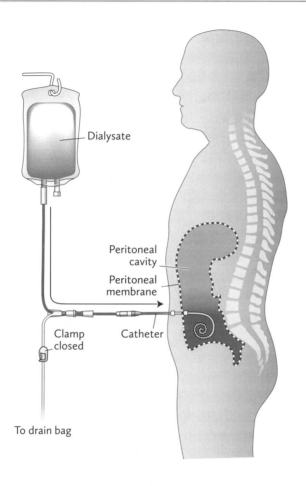

the catheter in place. With peritoneal dialysis it is crucial to avoid infections, which can occur because either the catheter or the exit site becomes contaminated. After the catheter has been in place for about two weeks, dialysis can begin. Once an exchange has been completed, a sterile cap with an antiseptic (like Betadine) on the inside is screwed onto the outside end of the catheter (on the left ends of the catheters in figure 6.4) until the next exchange.

FIGURE 6.4. Straight Catheter (*top*) and Curled Catheter (*bottom*) Used for Peritoneal Dialysis

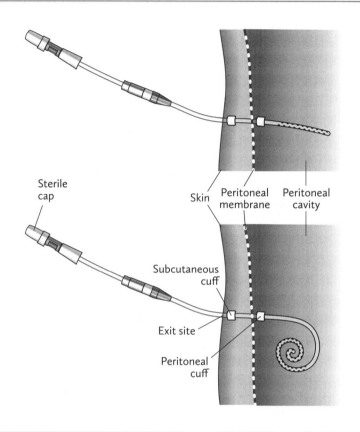

A surgeon has flexibility on where to place the catheter. Unfortunately, I did not talk with my surgeon about placement because I did not know that I could. As a result, when I received a peritoneal catheter, it was placed at my waistline. Wearing pants, with the subcutaneous and peritoneal cuffs directly under my belt, was very uncomfortable. Talk with your surgeon about what options he or she can provide for catheter placement that will minimize discomfort.

With patients who are obese, have an ostomy, prefer bathing in a tub rather than showering, or for children, there is the *prest-*

ernal placement. Instead of the abdomen, the catheter is placed in the chest and routed under the skin to the abdomen. According to Home Dialysis Central, evidence suggests that people with presternal catheters have fewer infections than those with abdominal ones.

Continuous Ambulatory Peritoneal Dialysis

To perform exchanges, you need good manual dexterity, but there are devices to help people with physical limitations. There are even devices that help blind people with exchanges.

Peritoneal dialysis is typically begun using a procedure known as *continuous ambulatory peritoneal dialysis* (CAPD), in which dialysis occurs throughout the day between changes of the dialysis solutions (called *exchanges*). Exchanging solutions is relatively simple—it is a process that takes about twenty minutes, once you are used to it. What follows is the description of a typical procedure for performing exchanges to give you an idea of what is involved.[3] (*Note: The following description is not a substitute for appropriate training by a qualified dialysis health care provider. Talk to your doctor or dialysis nurse about the best way to perform your exchanges. The supplies used in this description are provided by Baxter International. Fresenius Kidney Care also provides supplies for CAPD.*[4]) The exchange process must be sterile, so you must make every effort to avoid contamination. Hand washing with antibacterial soap or other suitable decontaminant is required at critical steps in the process. You may also want to dry your hands with a fresh paper towel rather than a cloth towel, to reduce possible contamination from the soiled cloth. Your dialysis center may provide you with an ultraviolet lamp to sterilize the connections between the tubing and your catheter.

Dialysis bags contain sterile solutions and come in sealed outer bags. After washing your hands, you will open the outer bag and remove its contents. Bags of dialysis solution include an attached drain bag, collectively known as a Y-set (figure 6.5). Before starting, warm the dialysis solution to body temperature (easily done in a microwave oven). Warm solution will help prevent abdominal cramping. Attach the fluid-filled bag to a bag pole and start your exchange.

After washing your hands and drying them with a paper towel, remove and discard the cap on the catheter. Then, attach the catheter to the system, which has a tube to the drain bag and one to the bag containing fresh dialysate. Before flow can occur, break two seals—one on the dialysis bag and one attached to the catheter. After allowing some dialysate to pass through the lines to prime

FIGURE 6.5. Y-Set Used in Dialysis

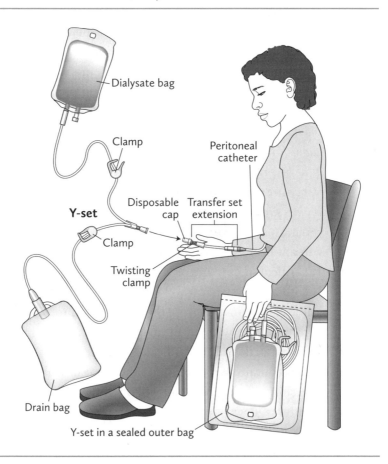

the system (the upper left side of figure 6.6), clamp the line to the dialysate bag and open the catheter line to allow drainage of your peritoneal fluid (the upper right side of figure 6.6).

Once drainage is complete, unclamp the line to the dialysate bag to allow flow of some fresh solution into the drain bag to remove bubbles (the lower left side of figure 6.6), clamp the tube to the drain bag, and then allow flow of fresh dialysate into your abdomen (the lower right side of figure 6.6). Because the force of gravity helps the dialysate to flow more easily, hang the bag above your head. When the bag is empty, clamp the tube from the dialysate bag and wash your hands again. Then, detach the catheter from the exchange system and immediately screw a fresh cap containing Betadine on the catheter. Finally, empty the drain bag and then discard the whole system. At this point, your exchange is complete.

Dialysis exchanges can be done almost anywhere you can find privacy. Avoid doing exchanges in public bathrooms or other places where there might be contamination. It is also best not to have people in the same room while you are exchanging—again, because of the risk of contamination.

If you work while on peritoneal dialysis, you will have to find a way to do exchanges in an office or comparable room. If there is a drop ceiling, you can attach the dialysate bags to the ceiling grid with an S-hook, like a plant holder. Otherwise, you may use a bag pole. During exchanges, you can continue working as long as you have privacy. To minimize the number of exchanges at work, do the first one as soon as you get up in the morning at home, one just before lunch at the office, one just before leaving for home at the end of the workday or when you first get home, and the last one just before going to bed.

This scenario may not work for everyone. For example, if you do not have your own office or another suitable place to perform exchanges, you may not be a candidate for CAPD. Continuous cyclic peritoneal dialysis may be a better alternative.

FIGURE 6.6. Dialysis Exchange with Peritoneal Dialysis

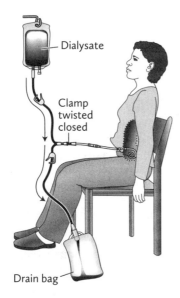

Dialysate

Clamp twisted closed

Drain bag

Prime the system

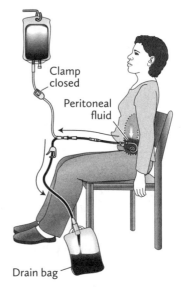

Clamp closed

Peritoneal fluid

Drain bag

Drain peritoneal fluid

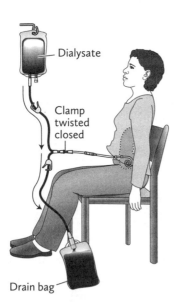

Dialysate

Clamp twisted closed

Drain bag

Remove bubbles

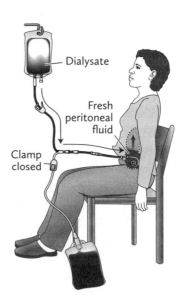

Dialysate

Fresh peritoneal fluid

Clamp closed

Replace peritoneal fluid

Continuous Cyclic Peritoneal Dialysis

Like CAPD, *continuous cyclic peritoneal dialysis* (CCPD) can be a useful option and requires training for a few days by a qualified dialysis professional. CCPD uses a machine, called a cycler, which performs exchanges during the night while you are asleep (figure 6.7). The machine (manufactured by Baxter International Inc. in Deerfield, IL) consists of several parts: (1) a dialysis bag heater, (2) a peristaltic pump inside the machine, (3) a place for a cassette (behind the door in figure 6.8), and (4) a computer (behind the control panel in figure 6.8) to run everything. The cassette controls the flow of fluid from dialysate bags to the abdomen and channels used dialysate to waste. All the tubing attached to the cassette is needed for dialysis (the disposable dialysis set in figure 6.9). The cassette works with the peristaltic pump to roll the fluids through the tubing. The computer is programmed to direct the flow either to waste or from one of the dialysis bags.

The rules for use of a cycler are similar to the rules for CAPD, especially when it comes to cleanliness. With practice and training on how the machine works and how to avoid contamination, you can set up the cycler for use in about ten minutes. First, place a 5-L or multiple 1-L dialysis bags on top of the cycler where the heater is located. Next, put the cassette in its receptacle and attach the drain line, routing it to a drain, such as a toilet, a sink, or a bathtub. Before attaching the appropriate tubes to the dialysis bags, wash your hands to avoid contaminating the bags when you insert the tubes. When the cycler has filled the tubing with fluid, wash your hands again, remove and discard the cap on your catheter, and then attach it to the tube at the far left of the organizer (figure 6.9).

Once the cycler is activated, you can go to sleep. While sleeping, if you turn more than once in succession in the same direction, you might become entangled in the tubing or crimp the tube. If this happens, an alarm will sound to awaken you, and the cycler will stop itself, as a safety measure. Train yourself to roll only back and forth when you want to change your sleeping position.

FIGURE 6.7. Cycler Used in Continuous Cyclic Peritoneal Dialysis

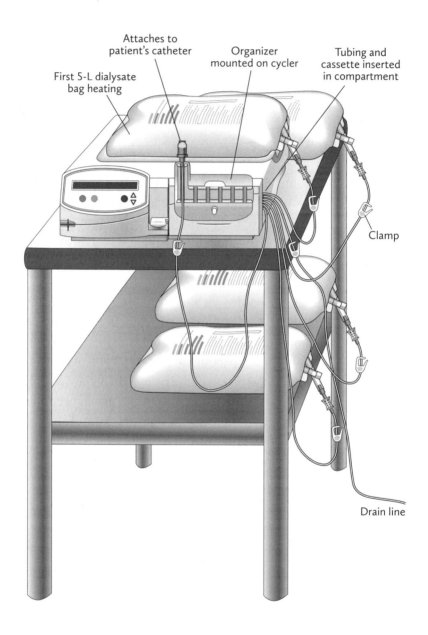

First 5-L dialysate bag heating

Attaches to patient's catheter

Organizer mounted on cycler

Tubing and cassette inserted in compartment

Clamp

Drain line

FIGURE 6.8. Parts of the Cycler

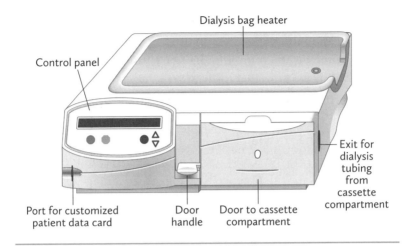

Dialysis bag heater

Control panel

Exit for
dialysis
tubing
from
cassette
compartment

Port for customized
patient data card

Door
handle

Door to cassette
compartment

FIGURE 6.9. Organizer and Tubing of the Cycler

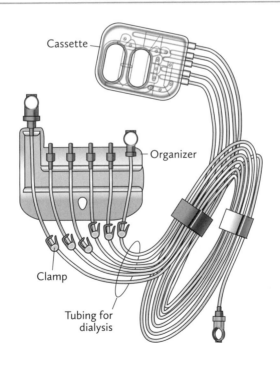

Cassette

Organizer

Clamp

Tubing for
dialysis

While you are asleep, the cycler does several exchanges as programmed on the computer, based on your nephrologist's prescription. As the amount of dialysate in the bag on the heater declines, the computer begins pumping dialysate from the other bags (if using multiple bags), so that the heater can warm the solution from those bags before use. After washing your hands the next morning, detach your catheter from the cycler and screw on a fresh cap containing Betadine. To complete the process, discard all the plastic tubing and the cassette. This process at first seems complicated, but it becomes less so with practice. The biggest advantage of CCPD is that fewer exchanges are needed during the day, especially if you still have some residual kidney function.

Monitoring the Effectiveness of Peritoneal Dialysis

Dialysis is a prescribed treatment and, as with other prescriptions, its effectiveness needs to be monitored. Nephrologists use two methods to determine how efficiently your treatment removes wastes from your blood. One test is the creatinine and urea clearance. This test is like the test your doctor requested to determine your kidney function before your kidneys failed (chapter 4). To have the test now, you will collect all the dialysis bags over a twenty-four-hour period as well as any urine you still produce in a large container. When you take the specimens in for analysis, you will be asked to provide a blood sample to determine how much creatinine and urea were removed from your blood.

Another way to measure the efficacy of your dialysis treatment is through a *peritoneal equilibrium test* (PET). In this test, you will be asked to provide a sample of dialysate at hourly intervals for up to four hours. The dialysate will be tested. The rate at which dialysis removes urea and creatinine from your blood and the extent to which your body absorbs sugar from the dialysate will tell your nephrologist how many exchanges you need to maximize the effectiveness of treatment. From this test, your nephrologist can determine whether your peritoneal membrane is a rapid transporter or a slow transporter. If it is a rapid transporter, your blood can more easily absorb glucose from the dialysate. This feature can make it difficult to maintain your blood sugar if you have diabetes; as a result, a person with diabetes needs more frequent exchanges. If your membrane is a slow transporter, however, you would benefit from fewer exchanges, with the dialysate remaining in your abdomen for a longer period.

Both CAPD and CCPD offer a great deal of freedom compared to hemodialysis. However, peritoneal dialysis may not be for everyone. Many nephrologists do not offer peritoneal dialysis as an option because some of their patients have developed *peritonitis* (an inflammation of the lining of the abdomen) from it. But peritoneal dialysis is worth considering if you have the discipline to keep up with all the exchanges and observe the routines necessary to maintain the required cleanliness. Your nephrologist will help you weigh the pros and cons of peritoneal dialysis (including peritonitis, covered later in this chapter) and will help you decide if peritoneal dialysis is right for you.

Hemodialysis

Hemodialysis works similar to peritoneal dialysis, except the blood is cycled outside the body through a special filter, called a *dialyzer*, by a machine usually located in a dialysis center (figure 6.10). Unlike peritoneal dialysis, which is a continuous form of dialysis, hemodialysis is intermittent. Thus, fluid, toxins, and electrolyte imbalances build up between sessions of hemodialysis, which means that the patient must restrict fluid intake and limit some foods. Most patients go to a center three times a week, with each dialysis session typically lasting three to four hours.

While some dialysis centers offer nocturnal hemodialysis, they increasingly offer home hemodialysis, but it accounts for only 1.9 percent of people being treated for kidney failure.[1] If you have someone who can help you or you can set up the machine, insert the needles into your fistula or graft, and monitor your session, home hemodialysis may be an attractive option, especially if you cannot schedule dialysis around work or if your center is not open late in the day. In addition to regular four-hour, three-day-a-week sessions, you may be a candidate for daily dialysis, which would reduce the accumulation of fluid and toxins between sessions. Home hemodialysis sessions last three to four hours each day, or they can be performed during the night while you sleep. Research suggests that daily hemodialysis may provide a better outcome than three-day-a-week, in-center sessions, because hemodialysis is more continuous. An increasing number of patients can dialyze at home, as long as their dialysis center can provide adequate

FIGURE 6.10. Dialyzer Used in Hemodialysis

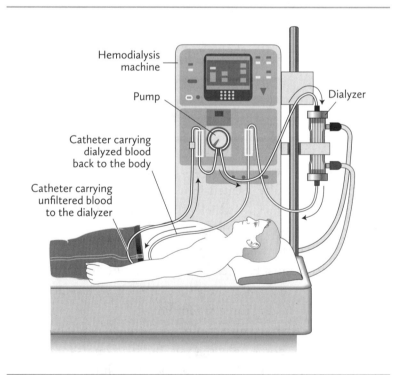

oversight and training either for you and/or a caregiver. To dialyze at home, you might need a person assisting you each time you dialyze, to monitor the treatment in case you experience bleeding or a drop in blood pressure, if you are unable to perform these tasks yourself. The latest generation of monitors sound an alarm if needles become dislodged. This alarm is especially important if you dialyze alone. If your center offers home hemodialysis, consult your nephrologist to see whether it is a good choice for you. More on the pros and cons of home hemodialysis later in this chapter.

The core of hemodialysis is the dialyzer, also known as an artificial kidney. The filter is composed of tiny filaments (semipermeable membranes) through which the blood passes (figure 6.11).

FIGURE 6.11. Filaments Comprising the Filter of the Dialyzer

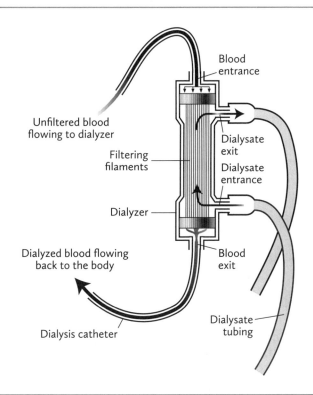

These filaments are bathed in a continuously flowing dialysate containing salts and buffers in concentrations that avoid excessive loss of these substances from the blood. This process in hemodialysis is analogous to the presence of dialysate in the abdomen when using peritoneal dialysis. The blood cells and large molecules pass through the dialyzer and return to the body, while the toxins flow freely through the pores in the filaments and wash away.

Vascular Accesses for Dialysis

If you are to receive hemodialysis on a regular basis, your nephrologist or a surgeon must perform a surgical procedure to access your blood supply; blood will be drawn, pumped through the dialysis machine and dialyzer, and then returned to your body. Typically, an access is placed when the estimated GFR (glomerular filtration rate) is below 20. With sufficient advance notice, most people can have a permanent access placed. Initially, however, it may be necessary to have a simple, temporary catheter placed in a large vein in your upper chest or groin. The two types of dialysis catheter are the untunneled (above the skin) and the tunneled (below the skin) cuffed catheter. Note that getting a vascular access can be problematic for those with poor circulation. This can include people with poor heart functioning and those with a life expectancy of less than six months.

If you need dialysis immediately, you may get an untunneled catheter placed through the right internal jugular vein in your neck into the right atrium of your heart or through the femoral vein in your groin. Your nephrologist, interventional radiologist, or surgeon will perform the procedure while you are under local anesthesia. You may experience a brief, temporary fluttering in your heart, if the tip of the catheter contacts heart muscle in the atrium. Untunneled catheters can be used only for a few days to a few weeks, because they tend to come loose, fall out, or become infected.

Tunneled, cuffed catheters may be used for a few weeks to a few months (figure 6.12). Buried under the skin, the tunneled catheter

FIGURE 6.12. Tunneled, Cuffed Hemodialysis Catheter

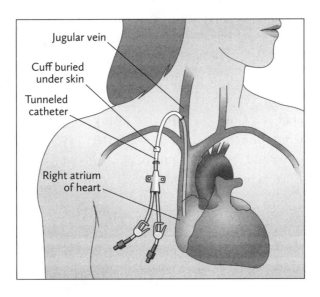

Jugular vein

Cuff buried
under skin

Tunneled
catheter

Right atrium
of heart

is larger and longer than an untunneled catheter and is less likely to be dislodged. Moreover, sealed against bacteria, it is less likely to become infected.

Neither of these temporary catheters will serve you for the long term, however. A more permanent and stable access is needed. Two types of access are used: the fistula and the graft. For both of these, the dialysis technician will insert two needles, one to draw blood into the dialysis tubing and one to return the blood. Both of them will provide a more efficient dialysis treatment than catheters, because the blood can be cleaned more quickly. Planning for a fistula or a graft should be done early to prepare for the time when dialysis will be needed. This is especially true because recent research has suggested that prolonged catheter use can lead to reduced survivals and problems with longer-term accesses.[5]

To create a *fistula*, a surgeon joins an artery in an arm or groin directly to a vein (figure 6.13). This procedure is done while you are under anesthesia. Over six to eight weeks, the pressure on the vessel increases, thickening the wall and then enlarging the vein, making it easier for a dialysis nurse or technician to place the large needles for dialysis. The fistula is the most desirable access to have. Because the fistula is created from your own tissues, it is more resistant to infection, lasts the longest, and has the least number of complications, compared to the other accesses.

The *graft* is a Gore-Tex tube that a surgeon places under the skin, attaching one end of the tube to an artery in your arm or groin and the other end to a vein (figure 6.14). In this way, the procedure is like the fistula procedure, and it, too, is done while you are under

FIGURE 6.13. Fistula Joining an Artery and a Vein

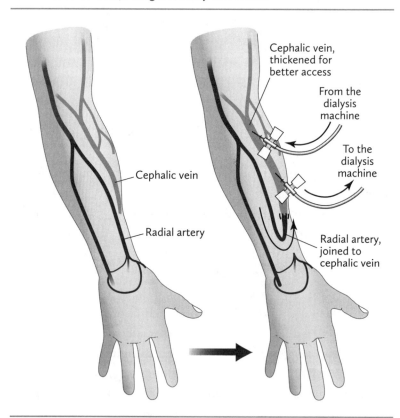

anesthesia. The graft may be used sooner than the fistula. Generally, you can use it after a two-week recovery period. Grafts are not as good as fistulas for dialysis and are more likely to become infected than fistulas. They are a good substitute if the veins are too small for creating a fistula, however.

Fistulas and grafts use needles with larger internal diameters than catheters, which allows the blood to move faster through the dialyzer; however, the access must be protected from excessive damage and infection. This is difficult to do when you're having dialysis three days a week, indefinitely. Keep the access clean and don't wear tight clothes around it. For the dialysis treatment, there

FIGURE 6.14. Graft Joining an Artery and a Vein

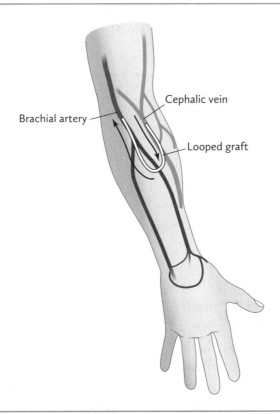

Cephalic vein

Brachial artery

Looped graft

is a way to avoid puncturing a fistula in many places. Using what is called the *buttonhole technique*, a dialysis technician or nurse can insert a blunt needle in the same spot every time, rather than using a different location with each session. Although there is a reduced pain with inserting needles in one spot, there is an increased risk of infection if the site is not properly cleaned.[6] If the buttonhole technique is not used, the injection site can be numbed using a local anesthetic prior to inserting the needles.

Dialysis is more efficient when blood can pass many times through the dialyzer during a session. To avoid clotting the access, the tubing, and the dialyzer, *heparin* (a blood thinner) may be injected into the access tubing. As a result, you may experience some bleeding from your access after dialysis. The staff in your center can minimize blood loss by applying pressure to the site using clamps. Some dialysis centers have special bandages containing a substance that helps clot blood.

Monitoring the Effectiveness of Hemodialysis

As with peritoneal dialysis, nephrologists must determine how effective hemodialysis treatments are. Nephrologists use two measures for this purpose: the *urea reduction rate* (URR) and the *Kt/V*. For the URR, the dialysis technician draws a blood sample from a port on the dialysis machine at the beginning and at the end of dialysis treatment and sends the blood samples to a lab to determine how much urea is in each sample. The URR is then calculated. A good URR is at least 0.68, which means that the treatment is removing at least 68 percent of urea from the blood.

Kt/V provides the best estimate of the effectiveness of your dialysis treatment. "K" stands for urea clearance during dialysis, "t" for time, and "V" for volume. The calculation of Kt/V is too technical to discuss here. Unlike the URR, Kt/V accounts for wide variations in weight among patients by determining the volume of water in the body and the nutritional status. Thus, the Kt/V provides a more accurate measure of effectiveness of a treatment. Good Kt/V values are at least 1.2 to 1.4. Using the Kt/V, a nephrologist can modify a prescription to maximize the efficiency of a dialysis session and help you feel better.

Your nephrologist has several ways to improve the quality of your treatment. For example, he can control the flow rate of your blood through the dialyzer. If you have a fistula or a graft, he can increase your flow rate to obtain more dialysis for your time at the center. Another way to improve your treatment is to increase the time on dialysis. Finally, with improvements over the past decade in the ability of dialyzers to remove larger-sized toxins, more options may be available to provide for a better outcome tailored to each patient.[7] As a result, your nephrologist not only can adjust time on dialysis and size of the dialyzer, but he can also order one to allow maximum purification of blood during each session, based on your specific medical situation.

Monitoring Your Health

Whether you are using peritoneal dialysis or hemodialysis, your health must be monitored closely. Your nephrologist will assess whether your dialysis prescription is optimal, and she will also help you stay as healthy as possible, so you can feel your best and participate in many of your regular activities. Your laboratory measures provide an open window into your health that will help your nephrologist treat you appropriately.

As we learned before, some of these measures still must be monitored. For example, urea (the BUN number on a lab report) and creatinine levels reveal how well dialysis is cleaning your blood. If these levels are too high, you may need to adjust your diet, or you may need to change your medications. Potassium levels are important in regulating heartbeat. If your potassium becomes too high, you could experience an irregular heartbeat or, in extreme cases, a heart block, resulting from a profound slowing of the heart rate. Calcium, phosphorus, and parathyroid hormone levels reflect your bone health. If phosphorus and parathyroid hormone levels are too high, you may have to limit further your phosphorus-rich foods or take higher doses of phosphate binders. Your nephrologist will also monitor your red blood cell count and iron levels. If you become anemic, you may require iron supplementation or erythropoietin injections.

There are other measures of your health. Albumin is a protein that can be a measure of your nutritional status. If albumin levels in the blood are too low, you will need to eat more calories and protein. Even if you are eating the recommended amounts of protein, you must consume enough calories from other sources, or your body will begin to burn protein for fuel. In addition, your nephrologist will assess your liver function as a general health measure and to look for toxicity from any of the medications that you take.

I recommend that you monitor and understand all your laboratory results. Your nephrologist or dialysis nurse can teach you the meaning of excessively higher or lower values and tell you about any treatment changes that might be required if the laboratory results change. Learn how to manage your diet, lifestyle, and compliance to your dialysis regimen. You may want to keep copies of the results to help you get a sense of what is optimal for you. All these steps will give you more control over your health and well-being.

Pros and Cons

Each type of dialysis has advantages and disadvantages. Talk to your nephrologist about these pros and cons to decide which type is best for you. If you have the opportunity, talk to other dialysis patients to get their perspective on which mode works best for them for their lifestyles, including work, family, and recreation. In general, people do as well on peritoneal dialysis as they do on hemodialysis. What follows are my impressions of the different dialysis modes based on my experience, as well as on information from other sources.

Peritoneal Dialysis

Only 7.1 percent of patients choose or can use peritoneal dialysis.[1] The main advantage of peritoneal dialysis is independence, because it does not require trips to a dialysis unit. Peritoneal dialysis works best if you are a self-starter, disciplined, and physically able to perform the necessary steps involved. Peritoneal dialysis is a better treatment than hemodialysis for people with low or unstable blood pressure (which can make hemodialysis difficult or even hazardous), a bad heart, or poor vascular access to the blood supply. Peritoneal dialysis gives you more control over when, where, and how exchanges are performed. Depending on your work situation, you may be able to dialyze in your office without interruption. Having a private space during exchanges can make peritoneal dialysis the more attractive option. You can even dialyze in the car if you have a long drive ahead of you. Avoid exchanges in public bathrooms or other places where contamination is a greater possibility.

Peritoneal dialysis also requires fewer dietary restrictions than hemodialysis. However, it is important to restrict your sodium intake to minimize fluid retention. Moreover, the body loses a lot of protein during peritoneal dialysis. You may need to take a protein supplement. One drawback of protein supplements is that many of them contain high levels of phosphorus, especially if they come from dairy products. One excellent option is powdered egg whites, sold by Optimum Nutrition (www.optimumnutrition.com), which taste good and mix well with water, milk, or juices. Also, buy the powder in five-pound containers. It is cheaper per serving. If you have diabetes, you may have trouble controlling your blood sugar with peritoneal dialysis, since the dialysate contains glucose. Talk to your nephrologist about the potential nutritional side effects of peritoneal dialysis.

If you like to travel or must travel often for your job, peritoneal dialysis may be preferable to hemodialysis. Dialysis bags and other treatment tools can be sent directly to your hotel. (Contact your equipment supplier in advance to arrange for delivery.) When traveling by plane, people who use CCPD can place the cycler in the overhead bins, if they are physically capable of handling a thirty-pound machine. Because checked luggage can be lost, it is a good idea to carry extra caps and tubing in your carry-on luggage. For travel within the United States, protections mandated by the Americans with Disabilities Act should allow a traveler to take a dialysis machine onboard the plane. In 2013, the US Department of Transportation ordered the airlines to transport portable dialysis machines for free under the Nondiscrimination on the Basis of Disability in Air Travel of the Air Carrier Access Act. This act covers items such as wheelchairs, portable oxygen tanks, respirators/ventilators, and canes. But with today's strict airport security procedures, you should double check with the Transportation Services Administration or your airline before traveling with your dialysis equipment. For international travel, contact the airlines.

There are some disadvantages that may dampen enthusiasm for peritoneal dialysis. Peritoneal dialysis can be time consuming and disruptive (although CCPD is less so). You must perform dialysis every day, regardless of your activities, although CCPD may require treatments only five to six days a week. Generally, you should be able to integrate exchanges into your life. However, depending on your work or travel schedule, you may have to arrange to do dialysis in the company of strangers, which you may find embarrassing. Occasionally, you may be forced by circumstances, for example, sitting on a plane, to skip an exchange, which is not a disaster if you rarely do so. Remember, you will feel your best if you perform all the exchanges that your nephrologist prescribes.

Although not as common as in the past, infections such as peritonitis are still possible. If you live in an area where the water supply comes from an unchlorinated well, or if you have any concerns about recurring infections and showers, whether using city or well water, you should consult your doctor for advice. Also, be diligent about cleaning your exit site using a sterile cotton swab dipped in a special bleach solution your dialysis nurse will provide. These precautions should minimize your chances of getting peritonitis. If you do get peritonitis, you might need to spend one or more days in the hospital getting treatment. Peritonitis is treatable, but if you have recurrent episodes, you may need to have your catheter removed. Infections can also occur at the exit site of your catheter. Again, it is important to properly clean the exit site regularly.

Peritoneal dialysis also causes weight gain and an increased waistline, which are mostly caused by fluid retention from eating too much salt. Thus, restricting salt intake is important. It may be difficult to find clothes that fit properly, because your abdomen may become quite large. This can lead to a poor body image. Moreover, you may feel uncomfortable with the dialysate pressing against your abdomen, especially if you have PKD and large kidneys. If you have PKD, abdominal hernias, ostomies, diverticular diseases, cancers in the abdomen, or leaks in your abdomen leading to breathing problems, peritoneal dialysis may not be a good choice for you. Leaks in the diaphragm can result in fluid in the lungs, in which case, you would have to switch to hemodialysis.

If your home has limited storage space, you may have trouble storing your boxes of dialysate and paraphernalia. In addition, carrying heavy bags of solutions can be difficult, especially if you are weak from the disease and have no one to help you daily. If you are single and live alone, peritoneal dialysis may not be for you.

Peritoneal dialysis also requires dealing with a considerable amount of waste. The empty boxes, some of which do not collapse, can create a special challenge if you do not have municipal curbside trash removal. Some people must transport their trash to a local disposal site. If you must haul your own trash, you will need to transport it more often, especially if you do not have a large vehicle. If you cannot remove your trash regularly, the amount of discarded material can become overwhelming. You may need help from your family or friends to manage the trash problem.

Finally, over time peritoneal dialysis can decrease in effectiveness. The peritoneal membrane loses its ability to extract toxins from the blood. When that happens, it would be necessary to change to hemodialysis.

Peritoneal dialysis offers many advantages if you prefer to be responsible for and manage your own treatment. Although it can be time consuming, peritoneal dialysis offers enough benefits that it may work well for you. Talk to your nephrologist and share your interests and concerns. She will be able to help you make a decision that will be best for you.

Hemodialysis

Hemodialysis has some advantages. For example, it is a good choice for people who like to spend time around other people. In addition, hemodialysis treatments provide structure and a consistent schedule to follow, with technicians at a center taking care of you. All you must do is show up, and the nurses and technicians do the rest.

Not all dialysis centers are of equal quality. I visited many in my travels while on dialysis, and they ranked from dreadful to outstanding. If you have the option, go visit as many centers in your area as you can. Distance from your home and easy transportation to them might be important to you. Look at the cleanliness, the arrangement of the chairs, and, most important, how the patients look. I have been to centers where the patients continually look sick and the center provided little comfort for them, such as pillows and blankets, sometimes not even lidocaine to reduce the pain of needle insertions. On the other extreme, I have seen happy patients with social activities and some exercise equipment to occupy their time. So, see if the staff is knowledgeable and if a social worker organizes activities for those who want them. Finally, check on available schedules to see if they work around your job. In addition, see if they offer home hemodialysis (more on that later in this chapter). Finally, check out ratings of dialysis centers provided by Medicare (www.medicare.gov/dialysisfacilitycompare). This will help with the selection process.

At hemodialysis centers, new patients often develop a sense of camaraderie with other patients and the technicians. Because you will be spending so much time with these people, it helps if everyone is on good terms. You may even develop some close relationships at the dialysis center, and they help pass the time. Some patients like talking, whereas others just prefer to sleep and be left alone. Or they watch television, read, or work on a laptop.

The disadvantages of hemodialysis are related to its advantages. Although people may prefer having a flexible schedule for their dialysis treatments, people with full-time jobs may not be able to schedule treatments easily. The stress of commuting, especially in a large metropolitan area, just adds to the difficulty of traveling to a dialysis center. For those living in rural communities, travel distances to a dialysis center may be long. Getting to and from a dialysis center can be a problem if you do not drive. Public transportation, taxicabs, and rideshares (Uber or Lyft) are options, and many people have relatives and friends who are happy to help with transportation. But caregivers run the risk of burning out while they try to help a loved one and find their own schedules becoming overburdened (see discussion later). The social worker at the dialysis center can assist you with finding suitable transportation if you need it. Otherwise, many people drive themselves. This can be risky because after a treatment patients are often dizzy from low blood pressure, nauseated, have a bleeding access, or cramps. I had problems with all of these issues when I was on hemodialysis. I can remember having to pull off to the side of the road, too dizzy to drive or needing to vomit. If these problems are excessive, your nephrologist may be able to adjust your prescription to help minimize them.

Medically, too, hemodialysis has a disadvantage that peritoneal dialysis does not have. As we saw previously, hemodialysis is an intermittent form of dialysis. Unlike peritoneal dialysis, which continuously dialyzes patients, hemodialysis allows waste products and imbalances in blood chemistries to accumulate between sessions. As a result, you will have to monitor your fluid, potassium, and phosphorus levels carefully. As with the peritoneal catheter, the access for hemodialysis may become infected.

Other disadvantages of hemodialysis involve the procedure. Because your vascular access, whether a fistula or a graft, is penetrated with needles, you may experience discomfort or pain. If you need it, ask the technician to use a local anesthetic, such as lidocaine. However, using the buttonhole technique for those with fistulas may minimize these effects.

During or after hemodialysis, you may develop cramps in your legs or feet, or you may feel lightheaded when you try to stand up. These symptoms are due to excess fluid removal during sessions, which is needed because you consumed too much fluid between sessions. The best solution is to restrict your fluid intake. Some dialysis centers will give you a salty solution to drink after a session. Although that helps at the time, you may feel thirstier and drink more fluid later. If you have difficulties restricting your fluid intake, talk to your dietitian about strategies to help you. Try to avoid having drinks close by or suck on ice chips instead when you are thirsty. I found not having drinks nearby to be a particularly useful strategy in restricting fluid intake. When working and keeping my mind otherwise engaged, I successfully kept my intake to 1 L per day.

Many patients complain about dry, itchy skin, called *uremic pruritus*. Not everyone experiences itching in the same way, which can occur on different parts of the body. Dry, itchy skin can be a result of several factors: dehydration, unmanaged phosphorus (more on this later in the chapter), insufficient dialysis, and allergies. Talk to your nephrologist to find ways to minimize this problem.

Complications related to the access may also develop over time, including clotting, infections, and bleeding. Your nephrologist can manage most of these side effects. If a fistula or a graft develops a blockage, then an interventional radiologist will be called in to remove the blockage. She will insert a catheter into the fistula or graft and attempt to dislodge the obstruction. If the blockage is a blood clot, the radiologist may use an enzyme called thrombin plasminogen activator (TPA) to dissolve it. Or she may insert a balloon, which can be inflated to enlarge the interior of the access site. Sometimes radiologists cannot repair the fistula or graft, and the patient will need a new access.

Many of the problems with in-center hemodialysis can be minimized by dialyzing at home. Home dialysis is becoming increasingly popular and is often recommended as the dialysis method of choice. If I ever had to go back on dialysis, home hemodialysis would be my first choice. Home hemodialysis has several advantages over in-center hemodialysis. They include improved survival, fewer cardiovascular effects such as better-controlled blood pressure, fewer dietary restrictions, better phosphorus and anemia control, improved sleep, and an enhanced quality of life.[8] It is often cost-effective if patients are reimbursed for their out-of-pocket expenses in addition to the equipment and other paraphernalia needed for dialysis.[9]

Doing hemodialysis at home is more complicated than in-center hemodialysis is. It requires a patient or a caregiver to learn how to set up the equipment and connect the patient to the machine. Patients can learn to "stick" themselves, if they are not squeamish. The training period is generally three to four weeks. The treatments can be done during the day, usually three to four hours a day, depending on the prescription, or at night. Nightly home hemodialysis can be tricky, if not dangerous, without a partner to monitor the situation. However, newer dialysis machines have alarms in case needles become dislodged, reducing the need for a partner.

Some barriers exist in parts of the world to people having access to home hemodialysis. Those who live in low- to middle-income countries or in less populated areas have the greatest difficulty in having access to home hemodialysis.[8] Even countries such as the United States have inequities in availability of home hemodialysis, especially among minority populations. With more and better resources directed toward these underserved areas, many patients with kidney failure might be saved. Home hemodialysis remains the most cost-effective way to provide hemodialysis.

A big advantage of home hemodialysis is fewer dietary restrictions to the point that they are like those of peritoneal dialysis. For those not able to do peritoneal dialysis, home hemodialysis provides an alternative that takes advantage of the benefits of peritoneal dialysis.

Conservative Care

When you are about to consider a treatment at a dialysis center, you are asked to sign a consent form. Usually, it will ask you to choose which dialysis modality you want to begin. It also has a choice of no treatment. When I saw that choice, I was startled because I did not expect it. I realized immediately that without treatment I would die from kidney failure. Living was a choice that fellow patients and I all had to make.

There are some people with kidney failure, however, who do not want to undergo the rigors of dialysis, because they are old and frail, feel that they have lived a good life, and it is time to let go. Often, these patients have severe complications with dialysis and have other chronic conditions, such as diabetes and high blood pressure. Besides, the process can be burdensome and remove them from their normal social and family interactions. Dialysis just is not worth it to them. This is a very hard discussion to have with loved ones. It can also be difficult for the doctors treating such patients.[10] After all, they want to save their patients and give them a good quality of life. Often, they question the patient's competence and try to convince the patient to start dialysis. Unfortunately, recent research shows that more than half of patients over age 75 die within a year after initiating dialysis.[11] On the other hand, there are options for those who really do not want dialysis. It is called conservative care or conservative treatment.

The goal is to make patients as comfortable as possible.[12] Efforts can be made to preserve kidney function and to treat symptoms such as nausea, pain, swelling, itchiness, and difficulties in breathing. It can also involve a strict diet, avoiding weight gain, and controlling blood pressure. Some people may want to try dialysis at home. In addition, there is a less intensive form of dialysis called, *palliative dialysis*, which keeps people alive longer but does not restore kidney function, that is, adequately remove toxins from the blood. Ultimately, this gives people time to continue life for a while and plan for end-of-life decisions. Regardless of the decision, it is for each of us to make in our own time and with our doctors and families.

Sleep Disturbances and Depression

Sleep disturbances are quite common in those with CKD. The most prevalent ones are sleep apnea and restless legs syndrome. *Sleep apnea* is characterized by a short cessation of breathing, lasting three to ten seconds, depending on the degree of blockage of the airways. *Restless legs syndrome*, a neurological disease with an unknown cause, is a strong and difficult-to-resist urge to move the legs.[13] Twenty to 70 percent of those with CKD experience some form of sleep disorder.

Among dialysis patients, 50 to 90 percent have experienced sleep apnea.[14] It can cause fatigue, cardiovascular events such as heart attacks and stroke, headaches, depression, and inability to think clearly. Sleep apnea can worsen kidney function, perhaps by activating the renin-angiotensin system, and exacerbating fluid overload. Standard treatment of sleep apnea is the use of a continuous positive airway pressure device (mask) that, when placed on the face, forces air into the lungs while the patient is sleeping. Other ways to reduce this problem is losing weight and avoiding sedatives and alcohol. Both nightly peritoneal and nightly hemodialysis can also help reduce sleep apnea.[13]

People undergoing hemodialysis may experience restless legs syndrome. Estimates of the percentage of people affected range from 12 to 25 percent of people who undergo hemodialysis.[14] Patients describe restless legs syndrome as creepy-crawly, itching, pulling, tugging, or gnawing sensations. These sensations begin when the person is at rest, not moving, and especially going to sleep. The symptoms of restless legs syndrome can be extremely unpleasant. You may have an uncontrollable urge to move and jerk your legs. If you resist it, the negative feelings may be overwhelming, almost painful. Moving may be the only way for the sensations to stop. Ultimately, you may get little sleep and feel exhausted during the day.

The mechanisms underlying restless legs syndrome are not completely known but appear to involve several neurotransmitters in the brain.[13] These include dopamine, serotonin, and glutamate. Restless legs syndrome disappears after a kidney transplant.

Treatments are available to relieve the symptoms of restless legs syndrome. To determine whether these treatments are right for you, your nephrologist will first examine your nutritional status. Deficiencies in iron and certain vitamins, such as B-12 and folate, can contribute to restless legs syndrome. However, since most people on dialysis take iron and vitamin supplements, nutrition is usually not the cause of restless legs syndrome for them.

Various medications can help relieve the symptoms of restless legs syndrome. For people with CKD, low doses of clonazepam (Klonopin), which is a benzodiazepine derivative with anticonvulsant, muscle relaxant, and anxiety-relieving properties, may provide relief. Other drugs in this same class may give you a hangover, however. Clonazepam works very well, even using the lowest dose needed to alleviate the symptoms. If you have restless legs syndrome, treatment with clonazepam may help you get a good night's sleep and feel rested during the day.

Anticonvulsants are another class of drugs your nephrologist may prescribe. Originally developed to treat Parkinson's disease, anticonvulsants like pramipexole (Mirapex) and ropinirole (Requip) may be helpful in treating restless legs syndrome. The downside is that anticonvulsant drugs can cause nausea, lightheadedness, and, in rare cases, hallucinations in some people taking these medications to treat Parkinson's disease. Since treating restless legs syndrome requires lower doses of these drugs than for Parkinson's disease, the side effects may not be as severe.

If you have restless legs syndrome, talk to your nephrologist. You do not have to suffer from this disorder.

Diet and Exercise

Fluid and dietary restrictions are more difficult to manage with in-center hemodialysis than they are with peritoneal dialysis and home hemodialysis. This is especially true for controlling sodium, potassium, and phosphorus.

Excess salt (sodium) retention (and therefore fluid retention) is often the most difficult to manage. Salt is in almost everything we eat, and sodium levels are especially high in processed foods and restaurant foods. Thus, knowing how much sodium you are consuming becomes critical. Here is what happens if you ingest too much salt.

The body uses salt (sodium chloride) to keep a balance between the volume of blood and the volume of fluid in the tissues. The proper balance is essential for healthy hydration. Ingesting too much salt has several consequences. Sodium draws water from cells in the bloodstream and into the tissues outside of cells. This can raise the volume of blood and can contribute to hypertension. The overfilled tissues swell, causing fluid retention in the legs and feet. In addition, excess fluid in and around the lungs can cause shortness of breath. Excess salt ingestion also stimulates thirst, which can lead a person to drink too much fluid, causing fluid overload in the body. You can minimize fluid retention by strictly controlling both your salt intake and your fluid intake. For some people, the nephrologist will establish a limit of 1 L (approximately 1 qt.) of fluids a day.

Potassium levels in the blood must be prevented from rising too high. The best way to control potassium levels is by restricting potassium in your diet. High potassium concentrations in the blood can lead to heart spasms and potentially death. Therefore, limit high-potassium foods, such as orange juice, bananas, tomato paste, potatoes, and colas. A complete list of foods to avoid is provided in table 6.1, and a list of foods low in potassium is shown in table 6.2.

High phosphorus levels have long-term implications—unlike high sodium and potassium levels, which pose more immediate concerns. As we learned in chapter 4, high phosphorus can lead to weakened bones and to the formation of plaques in various organs. Avoid foods high in phosphorus (table 6.3). Processed foods often have too much phosphorus. Although the new food labels now show potassium levels, they do not necessarily show phosphorus amounts. Take phosphate binders if your nephrologist prescribes them. Suggestions on how to substitute food with low phosphorus levels for foods with high levels are shown in table 6.4.

Read food labels to identify potentially harmful ingredients. Consider getting a nutritional guide to some of the foods you commonly eat. The American Association of Kidney Patients offers a free guide on their website, which includes sodium, potassium, phosphorus, protein, and caloric values (www.aakp.org).

TABLE 6.1 Foods with High Levels of Potassium

Fruits	Vegetables	Other Foods
Apricot, raw (2 medium), dried (5 halves)	Acorn squash	Bran/bran products
	Artichoke	Chocolate (1.5–2 oz.)
	Baked beans	Granola
Avocado (¼ whole)	Bamboo shoots	Milk, all types (1 cup)
Banana (½ whole)	Beets, fresh then boiled	Molasses (1 tbsp)
Cantaloupe		Nutritional supplements: Use only under the direction of doctor or dietitian
Dates (5 whole)	Black beans	
Dried fruits	Broccoli, cooked	
Figs, dried	Brussels sprouts	
Grapefruit juice	Butternut squash	Nuts and seeds (1 oz.)
Honeydew	Carrots, raw	Peanut butter (2 tbsp)
Kiwi (1 medium)	Chinese cabbage	Salt substitute/ "lite" salt
Mango (1 medium)	Dried beans and peas	
Nectarine (1 medium)	Greens, except kale	Salt-free broth
Orange (1 medium)	Hubbard squash	Snuff/chewing tobacco
Orange juice	Kohlrabi	
Papaya (½ whole)	Legumes	Yogurt
Pomegranate (1 whole)	Lentils	
Pomegranate juice	Mushrooms, canned	
Prunes	Parsnips	
Prune juice	Potatoes, white and sweet	
Raisins	Pumpkin	
	Refried beans	
	Rutabagas	
	Spinach, cooked	
	Tomatoes/tomato products	
	Vegetable juices	

Source: National Kidney Foundation website at www.kidney.org.

Note: Each item listed is a half-cup portion, unless otherwise stated, and contains 200 milligrams or more of potassium.

TABLE 6.2 Foods with Low Levels of Potassium

Fruits	Vegetables	Other Foods
Apple (1 medium)	Alfalfa sprouts	Bread and bread products (not whole grains)
Apple juice	Asparagus (6 spears)	
Applesauce	Beans, green or wax	
Apricots, canned in juice	Cabbage, green and red	Cake: angel, yellow
Blackberries	Carrots, cooked	Coffee (limit to 8 oz.)
Blueberries	Cauliflower	Cookies (no nuts or chocolate)
Cherries	Celery (1 stalk)	
Cranberries	Corn, fresh (½ ear), frozen (½ cup)	Noodles
Fruit cocktail		Pasta
Grape juice	Cucumber	Pies without chocolate or high-potassium fruits
Grapefruit (½ whole)	Eggplant	
Grapes	Kale	
Mandarin oranges	Lettuce	Rice
Peaches, fresh (1 small), canned (½ cup)	Mixed vegetables	Tea (limit to 16 oz.)
	Mushrooms, fresh	
Pears, fresh (1 small), canned (½ cup)	Okra	
	Onions	
Pineapple	Parsley	
Pineapple juice	Peas, green	
Plums (1 whole)	Peppers	
Raspberries	Radishes	
Strawberries	Rhubarb	
Tangerine (1 whole)	Water chestnuts, canned	
Watermelon (limit to 1 cup)	Watercress	
	Yellow squash	
	Zucchini squash	

Source: National Kidney Foundation website at www.kidney.org.

Note: Each item listed is a half-cup portion, unless otherwise stated, and contains less than 200 milligrams of potassium. If you eat higher amounts of an item than stated, you risk converting it into a high-potassium food.

TABLE 6.3 Foods with High Levels of Phosphorus

Beverages

Ale	Chocolate drinks	Drinks made with milk
Beer	Cocoa	
Canned iced teas	Dark colas	

Dairy Products

Cheese	Custard	Pudding
Cottage cheese	Ice cream	Yogurt
Cream soups	Milk	

Proteins

Beef liver	Crayfish	Oysters
Carp	Fish roe	Sardines
Chicken liver	Organ meats	

Vegetables (dried beans and peas)

Baked beans	Kidney beans	Pork and beans
Black beans	Lentils	Split peas
Chickpeas	Lima beans	Soybeans
Garbanzo beans	Northern beans	

Other Foods

Bran cereals	Nuts	Whole grain products
Brewer's yeast	Seeds	
Caramels	Wheat germ	

Source: National Kidney Foundation website at www.kidney.org.

Note: A high-phosphorus food generally has more than 100 milligrams per serving.

TABLE 6.4 Low-Phosphorus Substitutions for High-Phosphorus Foods

High-Phosphorus Foods (mg phosphorus)		Low-Phosphorus Substitutes (mg phosphorus)	
8 oz. milk	230	8 oz. nondairy creamer	100
		4 oz. milk	115
8 oz. cream soup made with milk	275	8 oz. cream soup made with water	90
1 oz. hard cheese	145	1 oz. cream cheese	30
½ cup ice cream	80	½ cup sherbet or 1 Popsicle	0
12 oz. can cola	55	12 oz. can of ginger ale or lemon soda	3
½ cup lima or pinto beans	100	½ cup mixed vegetables or green beans	35
½ cup custard or pudding made with milk	150	½ cup pudding or custard made with nondairy creamer	50
2 oz. peanuts	200	1½ cup light salt/low-fat popcorn	35
1½ oz. chocolate bar	125	1½ oz. hard candy, fruit flavors, or jelly beans	3
½ cup oatmeal	130	⅔ cup Cream of Wheat or grits	40

Source: National Kidney Foundation website at www.kidney.org.

You may feel overwhelmed at first by the list of dietary dos and don'ts. A dietitian can help you avoid the wrong foods, while showing you how to continue eating some of the foods you love. Restricting your diet may be difficult at first, but when you begin to feel so much better, you will decide it is worth it. Over time, tracking food values becomes second nature.

The healthier your diet is, the fewer complications you are likely to have. Eating right requires self-discipline and understanding from your family and friends, who must be sensitive to your dietary needs, since you may not be able to eat what they serve. At times, you may have cravings for foods that you should not eat. You may find that you can *occasionally* eat these foods but do so sparingly and in small quantities. You may find that you need only the taste of these foods to feel satisfied. Stick to your basic diet (chapter 5) and avoid forbidden foods and you will probably be okay. Be honest with your dietitian and nephrologist about what you are eating, especially if your blood chemistries are abnormal. They will be able to help you modify your diet to keep you healthy and allow you to eat some of the foods you like.

Hemodialysis is often associated with loss of muscle and bone mass, especially among women and the elderly.[15] This finding illustrates the importance of maintaining good nutrition and physical activity. Finding the right form of physical activity can be challenging, depending on your age and general health. Depending on the type of access for hemodialysis, you may have to be selective in the exercise you use. If you are mobile, walking is an easy and good exercise. It should not create problems with your access. If you do not have a catheter, gentle water aerobics is also an option. For maintaining muscle and bone mass, you normally would use weight-bearing exercises. In this case, light dumbbells with many repetitions could be beneficial. Heavier weights could be problematic if you carry too much fluid. Breathing could be difficult. In addition, it may be necessary to increase your protein intake to provide for good nutrition and support your muscle mass. Always clear any exercise program with your health care team to see what is most appropriate for you. Good nutrition can improve your overall health, including your muscle and bone density, physical performance, and quality of life.[16]

No one likes dialysis, and it is neither risk free nor complication free. However, it is possible to make dialysis tolerable and to limit how much it interferes with your activities. Talk about your options with your nephrologist and understand your own temperament and lifestyle. If you cannot obtain a transplant from a living donor before going on dialysis, then dialysis can provide you with a viable option for life while you wait for a transplant. In the meantime, help yourself by complying with your treatment, following your prescribed diet, restricting your fluid intake, and taking your medications. Taking care of yourself will make dialysis tolerable and will keep you in the best health possible.

A successful kidney transplant may be your best chance at living a long and healthy life. That's the topic of the following chapter.

CHAPTER 7

Transplantation

W E LIVE IN A CONSUMER SOCIETY. We buy things, and we throw things away, sometimes with little thought. But many people are developing a greater awareness that discarded items pile up in landfills, and as a result they are taking steps to recycle and reuse materials when they can.

Many people now view organ transplantation the same way. People who might otherwise die because of organ failure can live longer lives through *transplantation* of organs from living or deceased donors. Surgeons can transplant kidneys, livers, hearts, lungs, pancreases, intestines, bowels, bone, tendons, veins, corneas, and skin.

Organ transplantation has come a long way over the past forty years. In the early years of transplantation, doctors thought they could only transplant a viable organ from one person to another if the donor and the recipient were identical twins; otherwise, the recipient's body would reject the donated organ. Modern medicine has made major advances in the techniques of transplantation, and new drugs have been developed that suppress the body's normal reaction of rejecting a foreign body. How does transplantation work? How is it even possible? This chapter explores these questions and explains the transplantation process.

When medical science gained an understanding of how the immune system fights off foreign invaders, it was able to develop treatments to prevent organ rejection. Scientists used this knowledge to create vaccines to help the body destroy specific invading organisms such as those that cause polio. The vaccines helped the body produce proteins, called *antibodies*, which attack the invading organisms and cause their death. But even without a vaccination, the healthy immune system dispatches an army of cells to kill many bacteria, viruses, and other microorganisms it encounters that do not belong in our bodies. The healthy immune system is pretty amazing. But here's the downside for people who need transplants: because the body considers transplanted organs to be foreign, the immune system will attack them.

The body has an ingenious way of knowing what belongs to it and what does not: every cell in a person's body possesses a marker—a "name tag" of sorts—that distinguishes it from the cells in another person's body. When cells with different name tags bump into each other, a series of reactions occur, sometimes leading to the destruction of the cells that do not belong.

These name tags are known as *antigens*. Inside the body, cells called *lymphocytes* recognize whether the antigen belongs to you or to someone or something else. If your lymphocytes encounter recognizable cells, nothing happens. However, if your lymphocytes do not recognize a cell's antigens, the invading cells are killed. In the case of organ transplants, specialized lymphocytes called T-lymphocytes and a B-lymphocytes destroy the organ. When we talk about transplantation, we refer to the degree to which the cells are compatible with one another, and therefore the name tags relevant to transplants are called histocompatibility antigens, or human leukocyte antigens (HLA).

Your *HLA typing* and the HLA typing of the donor define how compatible a donor kidney may be.[1] Using the most recent methods of tissue typing, more than seventeen thousand types have been identified. In time, knowledge of these HLA types and small segments of antigen may lead to better matching. For now, cost and time of analysis prohibit its general use. In general clinical practice, at least five of the traditional histocompatibility antigens are used to determine compatibility for a kidney transplant from another person. These antigens come in more than one hundred forms and are not equally present in the population. Some are more common than others. The most common HLA antigens are present in about 20 percent of the population, whereas others are present in less than 1 percent of the population. In addition, some HLA antigens provide a stronger immune response than others do.

Until recently, for a transplant to succeed, these antigens had to be closely matched. Now, because researchers have developed more effective antirejection drugs, an antigen match is less important than it once was. A perfect match is still best, but less than perfect matches can be managed almost equally well with the latest immunosuppressant medications.

Are You a Candidate?

Kidney transplantation is the treatment of choice for kidney failure, allowing for the best quality of life. Your nephrologist will determine whether you are eligible to receive one. A kidney transplant is a serious operation, and living with a transplanted kidney requires lifelong care and commitment. Any donated organ is a valuable gift that must be given only to people who will take care of it. Therefore, you must take all prescribed medications, keep your doctors' appointments, and take care of yourself.

Your nephrologist can refer you to a transplant center who will assess whether you will be a responsible transplant recipient based on your previous behavior. If you are on dialysis, the transplant program will find out whether you came to the dialysis center for all your treatments (or performed all of your prescribed exchanges, if you are on peritoneal dialysis). In addition, it will check that you have taken all your medications and complied with any prescribed dietary restrictions. With a new kidney, your quality of life will improve, but that does not mean that your health is no longer an issue. After all, a transplant is not a cure for kidney failure; it is only a treatment. Thus, if your transplant team does not think that you will be compliant, they will not recommend you for a transplant.

Several other conditions can make it difficult to receive a transplant. Because the immune system will be deliberately suppressed with medications after a transplant, you cannot have an active infection or uncontrolled infectious disease, like a bacterial infection, at the time of the transplant. Failure of other organs, such as the liver, might make you ineligible. If you are HIV positive or have hepatitis B or C, you can receive a transplant and will do as well after transplantation as those without these infections. In addition, those with HIV and hepatitis C can be donors. In the case of HIV donors, their kidneys can be used only in those recipients with HIV. Those with hepatitis C now can be donors because the disease can be cured successfully in the recipients. To be eligible for a transplant, you should not have cancer or smoke, although those with cancer can be stabilized and evaluated again, depending on the cancer. Regarding smoking, centers may have different policies. If you have lung disease requiring long-term oxygen or heart disease that cannot be controlled, the transplant program may exclude you from getting a transplant. Evidence of drug or alcohol abuse will prevent you from getting a transplant until the problem has been resolved. Even obesity may exclude you from receiving a transplant, depending on the program, although obesity is becoming less problematic and can depend on other characteristics, such as age, underlying disease, gender, and race and ethnicity.[4] Although the policies of transplant centers vary, your potential longevity will be assessed to determine whether you would benefit from a transplant, especially if you do not have a living donor. The waiting time for a deceased donor may be years, so your likely future condition will be taken into consideration.

On a happier note, many people do qualify as transplant recipients. The prospect of receiving a transplant can be very exciting, especially if you have been on dialysis for a long time. Your ability to work, to engage in activities you love, and to just feel normal again will improve with a successful transplant. This chapter covers the steps you will take if transplantation is an option for you.

Donors

The number of people receiving kidney transplants has been steadily increasing since 1987. Ever since kidney transplantation began, there have been fewer kidney donors available than are needed (as we saw in chapter 1). As of March 25, 2021, according to the United Network of Organ Sharing (UNOS), over 91,100 candidates in the United States were waiting for kidney transplants (figure 7.1). Over the years, the number of people on the transplant list increased dramatically, peaking in 2014 at over 100,000 people. Since then, the number has declined leveling off in the lower to mid-90,000s. In 2020, 22,817 people received kidney transplants, slightly below 23,401 people in 2019, the highest number ever performed in the United States, and following an upward trend that started over the past five years (figure 7.2). This suggests that the number of transplants is beginning to catch up with the need, good news for those seeking a transplant. If the number of people donating continues to grow, the future could look more promising than it has in years.

Globally, transplantation is not universally available. As with dialysis (chapter 6), the ability to obtain a transplant varies based on socioeconomic conditions in a country. Most transplants are performed in the United States, Canada, Western Europe, Australia, and the Western Pacific Region, based on reporting from up to 115 countries.[2] Not surprisingly, funding for transplantation programs was highest in the most affluent countries, while funding was minimal in the poorest countries.[3]

Kidneys come from two types of donors: living donors and deceased donors. Not enough kidneys are available and acceptable for transplantation. This means long wait times for many

FIGURE 7.1. Number of Transplant Patients on Waiting List, 1998–2020. Data provided by the United Network of Organ Sharing and is current to January 1, 2020.

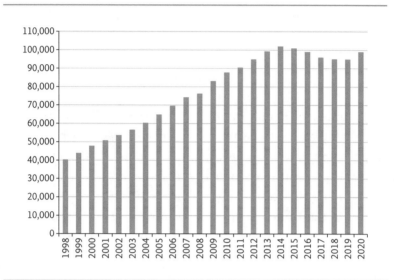

FIGURE 7.2. Number of Transplants by Donor Type, 1989–2020. Data provided by the United Network of Organ Sharing and is current to January 1, 2020.

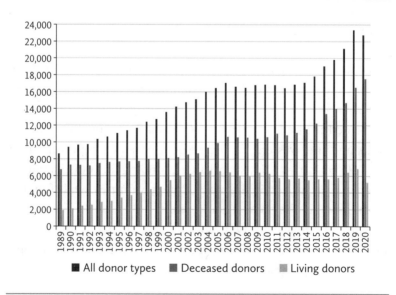

patients. This is especially true for people with type O blood, the most common blood type, because so many type O potential recipients exist for donations from type O donors. Survival rates for kidney recipients from both living and deceased donors are quite good and have significantly improved over the past ten years. One-year, three-year, and five-year kidney survival rates as well as patient survival rates for people who received a kidney from living donors versus those from deceased donors are displayed in table 7.1. (Kidney survival means living without dialysis or another transplant.) Patient survival is better than kidney survival, because patients may go back on dialysis after losing a kidney, while they wait for another transplant.

Another way to measure survival is using the half-life. The half-life is the time that represents 50 percent of those surviving kidneys that reach that point. The half-life of a kidney from a living donor is twenty to twenty-five years, while the half-life of a kidney from a deceased donor is eight to twelve years. Thus, half of people receiving a kidney from a living donor will still have that kidney functioning for twenty to twenty-five years, and half of people receiving a kidney from a deceased donor will still have that kidney functioning in eight to twelve years.

TABLE 7.1 Kidney Transplant Survival Rates

	Living Donor		Deceased Donor	
	Kidney	Patient	Kidney	Patient
1 year	97.5	98.8	93.2	96.3
3 years	92.5	96.1	85.1	91.3
5 years	85.6	92.1	74.4	83.3

Source: United Network for Organ Sharing (website at www.unos.org). Data are derived from transplants performed 2008–2015, compiled as of January 23, 2021.

Note: One-year survival is derived from 2012 to 2015 transplants, three-year survival in 2010 to 2013 transplants, and five-year survival in 2008 to 2011 transplants.

Living Donors

The public is more aware of the need for organ donations than ever before, and, as a result, more people are promising to donate their organs when they die. However, many organs are needed *now* to save the lives of people whose organs have failed. New interest in living donation has given hope to many patients in need of a kidney transplant. Since 1989, according to UNOS, the total number of living donations steadily increased, peaking in 2004. That number has been steady since then (figure 7.2). As a percentage of kidney transplants, living donations also increased, peaking at almost 43 percent in 2003 and then declining to 23 percent in 2020 (figure 7.3). The decline in living donations as a percentage of all kidney transplants is a result of more people willing to donate after death, as well as an increased availability of more usable organs from deceased donors, including those from the elderly for other older patients. Sadly, some of these organs may also come from those who have overdosed on opiates. Still, the increased awareness of living donation, including transplants from altruistic donors, and numerous ways to advertise for donors, has not significantly eased the shortage of kidneys from living donors.

Kidneys received from living donors generally have better success rates than those received from deceased donors. You may want to find a person willing to donate a kidney to you—although approaching someone about a living organ donation may be awkward. After all, you are asking someone to give up a body part and risk her own health with no medical benefit to her. Therefore, the gift must be truly altruistic. One approach to finding a donor is making your circumstances known to your family, friends, or groups in which you are involved. Those in need can solicit donors on social media sites such as Facebook. If someone is interested in donating a kidney to you, he or she will approach you.

Another source of donations is a kidney pool. In recent years, there has been an increase in the number of individuals donating kidneys to a nondirected pool of recipients through organizations

FIGURE 7.3. Percentage of Transplants by Donor Type, 1999–2020. Data provided by the United Network of Organ Sharing and is current to January 1, 2020.

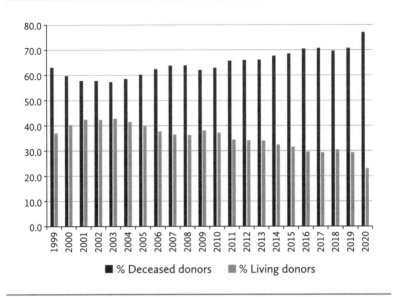

like the New England Program for Kidney Exchange, Matching Donors.com, and the National Kidney Registry ("Resources"). In donor pools like these, anonymous, or Good Samaritan donors do not specify the person receiving the transplant. To ensure that their gift is suitable, donors must be thoroughly screened and educated about the potential risks. Moreover, they must not be compensated for their donation, since cash payments for organ donations are illegal in the United States and in many other countries. If donations to a nondirected pool become more common, they could help relieve the imbalance between the number of organs available and the number of organs needed.

If you are tempted to buy a kidney abroad, do not do it! Studies have shown that people who do so generally have poorer outcomes. Because the donors *are* motivated by money, they may not be medically well screened. Medical tourism has become a flourishing business; marketing practices now include the temptation of exotic vacations coupled with a transplant from a living donor. Don't be fooled: *it is not worth the risk*. If you have a family member or friend living abroad willing to donate a kidney, however, that opportunity may be worth pursuing if the donor is thoroughly screened and if the kidney is a good match. Explore this possibility only through reputable transplant centers abroad. Talk to your local transplant center for advice.

Although many direct kidney donations from loved ones have good outcomes, a potential donor may not be compatible, usually because of an unacceptable blood type or a preexisting disease, such as polycystic kidney disease (PKD). To increase living donation, better methods have been devised to screen and match donors and recipients, so that more transplants might be possible ("Resources").

If you find a willing donor but that person is not a suitable match, you may be able to take advantage of a system of swapping, commonly called a paired kidney donation. Here is how it works. If you have an incompatible donor, your transplant center will try to locate another transplant candidate whose incompatible donor is compatible with you. If your donor is compatible with the other candidate, you can swap donors. If the second donor is not compatible with you, your transplant center may try to find other candidate-donor pairs in which one donor is compatible with you, and their incompatible donors are compatible with the other candidates. In such a case, a more complex candidate-donor swap can be performed. A Good Samaritan donor can even initiate a chain of donations if he or she is compatible with a candidate who does not have other compatible donors available.

With today's advances in removal and transfer of a kidney from a living person, most surgeons can remove a donor's kidney laparoscopically. In laparoscopic removal, the surgeon makes small incisions in the abdomen and then extracts the kidney through one of the incisions. The other incisions allow the surgeon to insert a video camera and surgical instruments. A minimally invasive laparoscopic operation means quicker recuperation for the donor than with traditional removal methods. These methods require an incision under the rib cage and can cause greater discomfort and longer recovery times.

When you are ready for a transplant, the transplant team will organize a meeting with your donor, whom you may or may not have already met, to explain the process and to answer any questions about living donation, the surgical procedure, and the short-term and long-term risks associated with a donation. These meetings may include family and friends. In cases of altruistic and swap donors, donor and patient may not meet at all. All information gathered about the patients and the procedure is confidential. Your transplant team may separate you and your donor for counseling and examination. Your donor will be seen by a nephrologist different from yours for the workup. Your donor and you will also have different surgeons. Medicare now requires that every program have a living donor advocate who is available to talk to your donor about concerns or reservations. Medicare and most medical insurance plans cover the cost of testing the donor for compatibility and the costs of the surgery.

Both you and your donor will undergo extensive physical examinations, be asked to provide your medical histories, and will undergo a battery of tests performed by your respective medical teams to ensure that your kidneys are compatible and that donating a kidney will not adversely affect the donor's health. In addition, your donor's nephrologist will make sure the donor does not have kidney disease and that he or she has two kidneys; the donor's nephrologist will rule out any infectious disease or cancer risk that the donated kidney may pose to you. If there are warning signs of potential pitfalls at any point in the process, your donor can opt out. This is especially true if the donor were in danger of a shortened life or medical problems in the future caused by the donation. The risks to the donor outweigh the benefits to the recipient.

The team will discuss with you, the recipient of a transplant, what is involved in your surgery, what will take place during the hospitalization, and what type of follow-up care you will need after you are discharged from the hospital. A crucial part of your after-care is the medications you will need to take to help your body resist rejecting your new kidney and becoming infected by various microorganisms. Therefore, the transplant team will discuss your ability to pay for your medications, which can be very expensive, to make sure that you have adequate insurance or other financial means to cover their costs. Medicare will cover most of the costs of medications for life after surgery. Even with Medicare, the costs are reimbursed 80 percent, unless the insured has drug coverage. Usually, there are copays.

In most cases, you and your donor usually must have compatible blood types. Because of the way we inherit blood types, some blood types are compatible, and some are not (table 7.2). For example, if you have type O and your donor has type A, B, or AB, your immune system will reject your donor's kidney. Thus, you both must have type O blood. On the other hand, if you have type A, B, or AB, you can accept a kidney from your donor not only if he or she has the same blood type, but also if he has type O. Type O is known as the universal donor. If you have type AB, you can accept your donor's kidney regardless of his blood type, making type AB a universal acceptor.

Some centers routinely transplant blood-incompatible candidates with comparable results as those with compatible blood types.[5] To prepare blood-incompatible recipients for transplant, the blood is cleaned of antibodies, depleted of B cells, and strong immunosuppression is employed. Type A also has two subtypes, type A1 and type A2. Some transplant centers can transplant a donor with type A2 into a type O without the need to clean the blood of antibodies. Before pursuing a blood-incompatible transplant, you should be sure that the transplant center is very experienced in performing them, and you should be sure that this is

TABLE 7.2 Blood-Type Compatibility

Donor	Candidate
A, O	A
B, O	B
A, B, AB, O	AB
O	O

the only way you can get a transplant. As discussed, you can get a transplant through swapping and through exchanges.

Other blood tests will assess your and your donor's general health and can reveal whether either of you has any active infections, including hepatitis or HIV/AIDS. An electrocardiogram (EKG) and stress test will be done to assess the activity and function of the heart to rule out underlying cardiac conditions that might endanger the health of you or your donor during or after surgery. Any condition that could harm your donor's remaining kidney, like high blood pressure or diabetes, would disqualify him as a candidate, unless he is low risk for developing cardiovascular disease. Finally, a social worker will conduct an interview with your donor to assess whether the kidney is being donated for the right reasons and not in exchange for payment or some other compensation.

Deceased Donors

Organs may also be obtained from a recently deceased person (cadaver). Not surprisingly, organs from deceased donors are more difficult to match to recipients than living donations are. With more people needing kidney transplants than there are kidneys available, the US government, through a contract with UNOS, has established what it believes is a fair and equitable procedure to allocate and match kidneys.

According to its website (www.unos.org), UNOS coordinates organ transplantations of all types with transplant centers throughout the United States. UNOS also coordinates multiple-organ transplants, such as kidney-pancreas and heart-lung. As of March 2021, UNOS maintained a database for all organs of almost 108,000 people needing an organ. UNOS oversaw over 39,000 transplants in 2020.

The UNOS database helps match organs from deceased donors to appropriate candidates. When kidneys become available, the organ procurement team removes them and sends information about the blood and tissue types by computer to UNOS, where staff members match potential candidates on the waiting list. Using the blood type, size of the organ, the patient's time on the waiting list, and medical urgency, as well as the geographic distance between the donor and patient, the computer generates a list of potential candidates.

The transplant coordinator in the transplant center then contacts the transplant surgeons caring for these patients. Each kidney has one primary recipient and at least one backup recipient. Because time is crucial, the transplant center may spend only one hour trying to contact the primary and backup candidates before UNOS goes to the other candidates on the waiting list. To minimize the time between recovering a kidney from a donor and placing it in a candidate, UNOS divides the United States into eleven regions (figure 7.4).

When a candidate on the waiting list matches perfectly with an available donor kidney, that candidate goes to the top of the national list regardless of how long he or she has been on the list. About 20 percent of transplants from deceased donors are a perfect match. When no candidate matches perfectly with the available donor kidney, UNOS offers the kidney first to a candidate with the next best match living in the same locality, and then living in the same region, before offering it to the rest of the country. Additional criteria apply (see later). Special consideration is given to those

FIGURE 7.4. The Eleven National Regions of the United Network of Organ Sharing

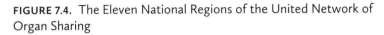

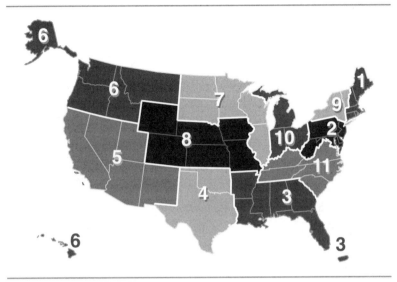

under 25 years old and highly sensitized individuals (those who have had previous transplants, transfusions, or pregnancies) because these conditions introduce foreign cells into the candidate, increasing the chances of rejection. Furthermore, some kidneys are transplanted along with a heart or a liver to the candidate when the person has kidney failure as well as severe heart or liver failure.

In 2014, UNOS initiated some additional or modified criteria for selecting recipients of a deceased donor. One changed criterion is the waiting time. It used to be time on the list. Now, it is time when a candidate's GFR ≤ 20 mL/min. or time on dialysis regardless of how long the candidate had been on the waiting list. This change gives those on dialysis a better chance of being transplanted sooner. Another major change is the concept of survival benefit. The idea is to match a donor and candidate that have similar characteristics, such as age. Young candidates are expected to have a greater chance of longevity than older candidates would. So, they would be matched with younger donors. This would especially pertain to matching donors who are children with candidates who are also children. Conversely, since they would not be expected to live as long as younger candidates, older candidates would be matched with older donors. Another change allows those who were living donors and who later in life develop kidney failure to move to the top of the list.

At this point, the potential match is given a series of scores, depending on the expected survival time of the donated kidney and the expected survival time of the recipient after transplant. Basically, the kidney with the longest functional expectancy would go to the potential recipient with the best chance of living the longest at the time of matching.

Although a candidate's chances of receiving a transplant improve with increasing time on dialysis, candidates do not actually occupy a specific slot. Ranking occurs only when a kidney becomes available. Historically, the primary consideration for a transplant depended on the extent to which the HLA type of the candidate matched the HLA type of a donor with the same blood type. Now, as previously discussed, a perfect match still goes to the top of the list, whereas with other kidneys, time when kidney failure began or time on dialysis is a predominant criterion.

Unlike candidates receiving transplants from living donors, where there are options for blood-type compatibility, an organ from a deceased donor must be an exact match. Requiring an exact match provides fairness for people with a specific blood type. Giving kidneys from donors with type O blood to people with other blood types, while possible, would create a greater shortage than exists now for type O candidates. This means an even longer wait time, currently the longest for all candidates. Therefore, it is usually not done. Once the blood type match is established, the cells from the deceased donor and from the candidate undergo further testing. There is one exception, however, to matching the blood type exactly. Some transplant programs will use kidneys from donors with type A1 and transplant them into recipients with type B.

Under the new allocation system, the survival benefit will help those with rare blood types, such as AB, and those with sensitized immune systems, such as those with a previous transplant that had failed. Candidates are given a score based on the degree of sensitization that is determined at the time a kidney becomes available and then given priority.

Before any transplant, laboratory tests will be done to assess the likelihood that the candidate's immune system will reject the transplanted organ. One test, the *panel reactive antibody* (PRA), measures the percentage of unacceptable antibodies in a candidate's blood that might react with a panel of HLA antigens found in the general population. It is a way of assessing the probability of acute rejection of any donor's kidney. With a high PRA, chances of rejection increase. These antibodies, which can sensitize a kidney to rejection, can be present because of previous transplants, blood transfusions, a disease such as lupus, or pregnancies.

The other test is the cytotoxic *crossmatch*, where lymphocytes from the deceased donor are mixed with the candidate's blood to determine whether antibodies are produced in the candidate's blood that could cause immediate rejection of the kidney. A positive crossmatch indicates certain rejection. Thus, a *negative* crossmatch is desired. Once these criteria have been satisfied, the transplant surgery can proceed.

Waiting for a Transplant

The wait for a kidney transplant can be frustrating and can seem endless.[6] Many people with kidney failure decide to get a kidney transplant rather than start or continue dialysis. After undergoing all the extensive tests and finally being placed on the transplant list, the wait begins. For a lucky few, the wait is short. Some people receive transplants within months. However, most people wait years for a transplant. For people who have not found a compatible kidney from a living donor, the wait is about three to seven years. Wait times also vary depending on where in the country a candidate lives. I was on the list for more than seven years, and the wait was often difficult.

When I first started dialysis in 1997, I was quite ill. I didn't think much about transplantation until I became well enough to consider it. Then my biggest concern was being unavailable to my transplant coordinator who could call at any time to say, "It's time." Like many people on the wait list, I carried a cell phone; I also always had a pager with me (cell phones were new at the time, and cell coverage was limited and poor at sending signals indoors), not knowing whether I would receive a signal when I was in a large building or far away from home.

The longer I was on the transplant list, the less I wanted to travel very far from home. Wherever I went, I made sure the transplant coordinator knew where I was and how she could contact me. Even so, I was always concerned about receiving a call or returning in time to receive my kidney. Although a surgeon can effectively transplant a kidney within twenty-four hours (at the time), the chances that the kidney will function immediately decrease with increasing time after removal from the donor. Consequently, I lived in fear that I would miss that great gift of life by being in the wrong place at the right time.

Those of us on the transplant list know that we have limited ability to plan for the day the transplant coordinator calls. We could have a bag packed and have family and friends ready to help, but we do not know for sure if our plans will work. It is not as if we know exactly when our transplant will happen. Over the seven and a half years I lived with dialysis, although I often found myself becoming increasingly anxious about my availability for a transplant, all I could do was stay in contact with the hospital, hang in there, live my life the best way I could, and wait. Although patience may be a virtue, at times I found it hard to maintain. At some point, we need faith that, in the end, everything will work out. We will receive our transplant, and our lives will improve. I received my transplant on January 2, 2005.

Having a Transplant

When the time comes for your transplant, it is often a surprise. Many candidates waiting for transplants receive numerous calls that do not pan out. Because UNOS does not know for sure whether the primary candidates are available, many candidates receive calls as possible backups to determine their readiness. Eventually, you will percolate to the top of the list and finally get your call as a primary candidate.

Once you receive the call and accept the organ, you will go to the transplant center to prepare for surgery. The center will perform blood tests to make sure your health is good enough for the transplant surgery to proceed. Part of waiting for surgery involves the time to transport the kidney to the center and to complete the crossmatch to ensure that you will not reject your new kidney immediately. As one of the final preparations for surgery, a nurse will insert a catheter into a vein, and the anesthesiologist will begin administering sedatives. Once you are in the operating room, the anesthesiologist will give you general anesthesia.

The transplant itself, whether the kidney comes from a living or deceased donor, is relatively simple, as figure 7.5 illustrates. In living donations, left kidneys are transplanted because they have longer *ureters* (the long tubes connecting the kidney to the bladder) than right kidneys. In deceased donations, either kidney may be used. The organ procurement surgeon dissects the kidney from the deceased donor and its attachments from its surroundings. The kidney is immediately perfused with a preservation solution composed of high potassium and other nutrients and is cooled down to decrease oxygen demand; these steps keep the kidney as healthy as possible. In the operating room, your transplant surgeon will place the kidney into your lower abdomen. He or she will attach the blood vessels of the new kidney to the external iliac artery and vein in the groin and then attach the new ureter to the bladder. During the operation, the surgeon will insert a Foley catheter into the urethra to the bladder to collect urine. The native kidneys are not usually removed unless they are chronically infected, as in PKD patients with infected cysts or unusually large kidneys, although they may be removed safely at the time of transplant.[7] Otherwise, they don't normally pose a threat to the patient.

FIGURE 7.5. The New Kidney in Place after the Transplant Procedure. The transplanted kidney on the right side of the body appears on the left in the figure, which is facing us.

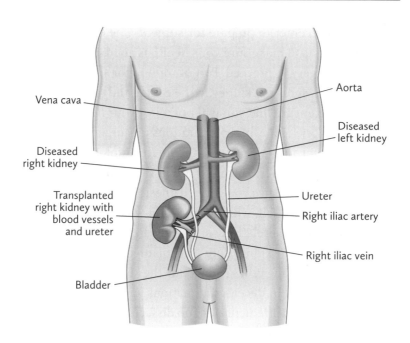

Postoperative Care

After the three- to four-hour transplant operation, proper care and monitoring becomes essential to manage postoperative pain, to prevent rejection of your kidney, and to minimize infections. Your recovery in the hospital will last, on average, five to seven days, during which time you will receive numerous medications to control the aftereffects listed earlier. Initially, your immune system must be heavily suppressed with antirejection medications, which reduce the likelihood of rejecting the organ but increase the likelihood of contracting infections. To counteract this possibility, you will receive antibiotic, antiviral, and antifungal agents to reduce the chances of infection. You must take these medications exactly as prescribed. Before the transplant you will have told your transplant team about any other medications you are taking, and the team will adjust your medications to avoid potentially serious drug interactions.

Once you are released from the hospital, you must keep daily records of your blood pressure, temperature, fluid intake, and urine output and have your blood tested regularly to detect the possibility of infection or kidney rejection. You must also eat a healthy diet and exercise regularly once your incision has healed. A healthy lifestyle is essential during the first year (and beyond) to keep your body in the best shape possible. The post-transplant coordinator at the center will outline the regimen you must follow. The need for blood tests diminishes over time, as your body accepts the new kidney.

Taking immunosuppressants over the longer term is the cornerstone of treatment to prevent rejection of your newly transplanted kidney. Your transplant surgeon, depending on the center's protocol and experience, can prescribe several different drugs. Before and immediately after the transplant, intravenous medications such as anti-thymocyte globulin (Thymoglobulin) and basiliximab (Simulect) may be administered to reduce the chances of rejection. The main antirejection medications currently prescribed for long-term use are steroids—prednisone (Deltazone) and methyl-prednisolone (Medrol) and other types of antirejection medications, such as tacrolimus (Prograf), sirolimus (Rapamune, Rapamycin), mycophenolate mofetil (Cellcept), mycophenlic acid (Myfortic), cyclosporine (Neoral, Gengraf), and the newer belatacept (Nulojix). Cheaper generic medications are available and used routinely.

Less than 10 percent of transplant recipients experience acute rejection during the first six months post-transplant. However, with time, as the body accepts the kidney, the doses of immunosuppressants will be reduced to maintenance doses. If you experience acute rejection, as determined with a kidney biopsy, the treatment depends on whether the rejection is caused by T-cells or antibodies.[8] For T-cell-mediated rejection, short-term treatment with steroids or thymoglobulin are used, whereas for antibody-mediated rejection, cleansing the plasma of antibodies is an option. In addition, adjustments will be made to the maintenance doses of your immunosuppressant drugs. If acute rejection occurs numerous times, the kidney may undergo chronic rejection by the body, which can lead to the loss of function over the long term.

New advances in the treatment of hepatitis C brings new opportunities for transplantation for those with hepatitis C infections. New combination antiviral therapies have shown promise in completely curing the disease and allowing hepatitis C patients an opportunity to be transplanted with hepatitis C–infected kidneys.[9] Moreover, this advance can increase the pool of donors for recipients who do not have the disease. Indeed, noninfected candidates have been transplanted with infected kidneys and then treated with a combination of antiviral drugs.[10] Clinical trials are ongoing to test this treatment further.

Immunosuppressant drugs have many side effects. Because they suppress the immune system to prevent rejection, the body becomes more prone to infections of all types, including bacterial, viral, and fungal infections. During the first six months after transplant, immunosuppression is at its highest level. To reduce the risk of infection during this time, doctors will prescribe separate drugs for each threat, such as sulfamethoxazole/trimethoprim (Bactrim) for bacterial infections that include pneumonia, acyclovir (Zovirax) for viral infections such as herpes, valganciclovir (Valcyte) for cytomegalovirus (CMV), and clotrimazole troche (Mycelex) for fungi, especially of the mouth and throat. If you have no infections after six months, your surgeon will discontinue these medications.

Immunosuppressants may increase your risk of developing cancer, especially lymphoma. People taking immunosuppressants are also at a higher risk of developing skin cancers. Careful monitoring is required to detect cancer early and to initiate early treatment. You will need regularly scheduled diagnostic tests such as mammograms, PAP smears, colonoscopies, and skin cancer screens to prevent cancers from developing out of control.

Another side effect of antirejection medications is developing elevated blood lipids (*hyperlipidemia*), which are higher than normal values for cholesterol and triglycerides in the blood. Elevated cholesterol and triglycerides are risk factors for heart disease and stroke. If you have elevated blood lipids, you will need to take atorvastatin (Lipitor), simvastatin (Zocor), or fenofibrate (Tricor). In addition, you must eat a low-fat diet.

Immunosuppressant drugs pose additional complications for transplant patients. As we have seen throughout this book, diabetes is the major cause of kidney failure. Unfortunately, tacrolimus can complicate management of type 2 diabetes. Steroids may increase your risk of developing osteoporosis. Osteoporosis results from the loss of calcium from the bones, making them more brittle and prone to fracture. If you have been on dialysis, you are probably familiar with this risk, which steroids may only increase. Fortunately, many transplant centers are lowering steroid doses as much as possible.

Many people awaiting a transplant have high blood pressure. After a transplant, it is common for blood pressure levels to decline dramatically. However, some immunosuppressants can elevate blood pressure, as well as increase the risk for cardiovascular disease. Your center will closely monitor your blood pressure for any sudden increases or decreases.

Weight gain is a common problem with those receiving a transplant. In some cases, the weight gain can be as much as one hundred pounds. This is caused by the immunosuppressant medications. Not only do some of them lead to fluid retention, but they can also inhibit the ability of the body to burn fat deposits. Although you will be able to eat whatever foods you like, you may find that you will have to limit your caloric intake. I have had this problem since I had my transplant. To deal with weight gain, in addition to limiting my food intake, I engage in a rigorous, daily exercise program, consisting of strength training and aerobics (CrossFit) that keeps my weight under control. As an added benefit, this program has also kept my blood pressure and blood glucose levels under control without medications. Before you start such an exercise program, consult your transplant team to ensure that you are physically able to do it.

Because the functioning of one transplanted kidney will never be equivalent to two normal kidneys, your creatinine, blood urea nitrogen (BUN), and GFR will be monitored. If kidney function begins to deteriorate after many years, your nephrologist will assess whether any of the health problems that you experienced before your transplant, such as anemia and bone disease (chapter 4), resemble the current decline, and then treat you accordingly.

Despite potential complications after transplant, with a new kidney you can expect a considerable improvement in your quality of life. You should have no problem working, traveling, and engaging in the activities that you enjoy. You may find, as many transplant recipients do, that receiving a kidney transplant is like being born again. You will feel so much better that in time you may forget the worst experiences of CKD. Life will be yours for the taking, but only *if you care for your new kidney and follow all the instructions of your transplant team.* Remember, a kidney transplant is not a cure but a treatment.

Diet after Transplant

Throughout this book, I have described many challenges that those of you with CKD and kidney failure have had with what you can eat. As you progressed through the stages of kidney failure, more and more restrictions on diet were usually needed. By the time you were on dialysis, considerable restrictions, especially in potassium and phosphorus intake, or needing to eat enough calories and protein were required. Now, the good news! After a kidney transplant and recovery, restrictions normally are lifted. Generally, you can eat whatever you want, consistent with a healthy diet. Be sure to consult your transplant team to ensure that you do not change your diet too quickly. For me, it was life changing. To be able to eat the foods I missed was glorious. One problem I had though in adapting to a normal diet was eating enough salt. Being so restricted, especially while on dialysis, often I became dehydrated after being transplanted. I even had to begin salting my food to retain the fluid that I drank. Small matter. Having the freedom to eat what I missed was exceptionally satisfying. You may also enjoy your newfound freedom. Enjoy!

Clinical Trials

Participating in a clinical trial is one route to receiving a transplant. Clinical trials are research projects using human subjects and are designed to answer specific health questions. Most trials assess whether a new medication or procedure will be an effective treatment for patients with a specific disease. In the case of kidney transplants and the disease requiring them, numerous clinical trials are under way. To learn more about them, visit the National Institutes of Health (NIH) Clinical Trials website (www.clinicaltrials.gov).

I became interested in clinical trials more than a year before I received my kidney transplant when I realized that getting a new kidney might not be the end of living with kidney failure. I could be unlucky and lose my kidney to rejection or infection. I also knew what long-term use of immunosuppressant drugs could do to my body, especially steroids. Therefore, I decided to focus on finding ways to maximize the long-term success of my new kidney and to reduce the possible complications induced by these drugs by possibly enrolling in a clinical trial designed to do just that.

After talking to my transplant coordinator and the social worker at my dialysis center, I learned that NIH had ongoing clinical trials that matched my interest. I called the transplant coordinator at NIH and told her of my interest in participating in a trial. After thoroughly reading the research protocols, I made an appointment to meet with the transplant coordinator and the principal investigator.

The goal of my first visit was to gather information about the program and the credentials of the researchers. Being a researcher myself, I wanted to delve into the scientific rationale of their research, their accomplishments and disappointments with their results, and the possible risks of enrolling in the trial. I scoured the publications that they provided.

The science behind their research and the trial made a great deal of sense to me. The researchers designed the protocol to make the body tolerant to the presence of a foreign organ, thereby reducing the likelihood of rejection. In doing so, a transplant recipient would need fewer immunosuppressant drugs and no steroids to avoid rejection. As to risk, they had lost no kidneys due to rejection since NIH established their transplant institute in 1999. Only two kidneys were lost because of viral infections.

Knowing these statistics, I decided that I could accept the risks and that the clinical trial was worth considering seriously. From what the doctors told me, I was convinced that participating in the trial would not adversely affect my outcome, compared to standard care at a traditional transplant center. As additional insurance, I asked my nephrologist to call the principal investigator, who was also the transplant surgeon, to assess for herself the potential risks

I would be taking. After talking to the surgeon, my nephrologist felt that I would not be taking any additional risks if I participated. After doing my own research and with the support of my nephrologist, I decided to enroll in the study and did not look back. My preparation for the transplant mirrored that described earlier in this chapter.

More than sixteen years have passed since my transplant, and I have experienced no rejection episodes and no significant infections. I am currently taking a small dose of only one immunosuppressant drug. Moreover, I no longer have high blood pressure. As a result of living a healthy lifestyle, I have been able to travel all over the world, which is what I enjoy doing.

After participating in this clinical trial, I arrived at several conclusions about the benefits and drawbacks of clinical trials, and I have some ideas about how to decide whether to participate in one. Here are some issues to consider.

How Far Along Is the Research?

Clinical trials progress in several phases based on the number of subjects and the questions asked. Phase 1 trials tend to have fewer participants and are designed to determine the safety of the medication and range of doses for use in future trials. If the medication is new, with few studies done in humans, the greatest risk could occur during Phase 1 trials. Other Phase 1 trials are designed to test drugs approved by the Food and Drug Administration (FDA) for one application, but researchers want to evaluate their use for a new one, perhaps for a disease for which the medication was not originally intended, known as *repurposing* (chapter 8). In this case, participation in a Phase 1 trial is less risky because much of the drug safety testing has already been done.

Phase 2 trials enroll more subjects, typically a few hundred. At this stage, efficacy and safety become important factors. I chose to participate in a Phase 2 trial because the experimental drugs had already been FDA approved for another application. In addition, the researchers had good evidence that the protocol had a high chance of success.

Phase 3 trials may involve thousands of patients and are conducted in multiple centers around the country and even the world. By this point, safety and efficacy have been reasonably established. The risks are substantially reduced, but death or less severe complications may occur in a small percentage of participants.

Understanding the Protocol

Scientific research is often difficult to understand, especially for people who do not have training in science. The scientific jargon can sound like a foreign language. Although I understood much of it, there were terms and research issues that were unfamiliar. Anyone participating in a clinical trial has the right to understand fully what the study involves and what risks are possible. Keep asking questions until you are satisfied that you understand all the potential risks and rewards. If necessary, ask your doctors for help. I found that my nephrologist's input helped allay any remaining concerns I had about enrolling.

Advancing Medical Research

Many people decide to enroll in a clinical trial because conventional means of treatment have not been successful. Their participation in a clinical trial may be their only hope for survival. Good candidates for kidney transplants typically do not face this dilemma. Standard transplant protocols are acceptable and are generally preferable to remaining on dialysis.

Even in clinical trials, the use of medications or procedures occurs only after rigorous research, first with experimental animals and then with human subjects. To advance this research, human volunteers are needed. If people did not participate in clinical trials, there would be no new drugs! People who participate in clinical trials realize that they are making a significant contribution to improving the health of their fellow humans and perhaps themselves, too. The prospect of making a difference gave me considerable satisfaction. I had worked in medical research for more than forty years, and my participation gave me an opportunity to continue contributing. You may feel the same way.

Medical Insurance and Care

Another benefit of enrolling in a clinical trial is cost. People who enroll in a trial receive free treatment and health care relevant to the study, which may be especially attractive for people who do not have medical insurance. Although Medicare will cover much of the cost of a transplant, the remaining costs can still be substantial. A transplant recipient can save a considerable amount of money, especially for prescription drugs, by participating in a trial. Even though I had a good health insurance policy, participating in the clinical trial still saved me money.

My Experience

My transplant surgeon called me at 3:30 one morning to tell me that my time had come to receive a new kidney. I was happy yet apprehensive about what to expect. Even though I had prepared for this day, now the idea of a transplant changed from the abstract to a reality.

At 6:30 a.m., I drove to NIH, where for several more hours I waited for the lab to complete the final testing to make sure I was compatible with the kidney. At about 11 a.m., the nurse placed an intravenous line into my arm and gave me a sedative. As the nurses wheeled me to the operating room, the sedatives must have kicked in, because I do not recall getting there. I awoke several hours later in the recovery area with a new kidney.

For me, the immediate postoperative issues were recovering from the anesthesia and managing pain. I find general anesthesia disorienting. In the past, I have had visual and sometimes auditory hallucinations for several days after receiving general anesthesia. Although I found this disconcerting, I knew that they would go away. An additional complication for me was getting my bowels to function properly, which took several days. Pain can be managed with a morphine drip or by self-administration using a pump, which controls the amount, maximum dose, and appropriate intervals of intake. (Morphine, unfortunately, tends to cause constipation, which further complicates the bowel problem.) Thanks to a morphine drip, I had no significant postoperative pain, even though I had an eight-inch incision in my lower abdomen.

As part of the clinical trial, I received a medication just after my transplant to further reduce my chances of rejecting my kidney. In addition to antirejection medications, my doctors prescribed antithymocyte globulin (Thymoglobulin) for several days to deplete the T-cells responsible for rejection. This treatment kept my T-cell count low for almost two weeks. In the program's experience, the immune systems of patients given antithymocyte globulin were less responsive to a foreign kidney, compared to a standard treatment protocol. For me, antithymocyte globulin had a strange side effect. My hands itched, and then the skin peeled. They were unsightly for a while but returned to normal after the last dose of the drug.

Before transplant, my high blood pressure was difficult to control, even with high doses of three different blood pressure medications. After my transplant, my blood pressure dropped to the point where I needed only one medication. After six months, I no longer needed any blood pressure medication at all. Normal blood pressure was a major benefit of having a kidney transplant.

Like many people receiving kidney transplants, I had elevated blood lipids before receiving my transplant. In fact, my blood lipids were initially so high after my transplant that the nurse who drew my blood could see the fat in the sample. It was fortunate that I did not have a heart attack or stroke. At the time, I was taking sirolimus and tacrolimus as my antirejection medications. To treat the high blood lipids, my doctors took me off the sirolimus, which was identified as the cause. With proper treatment—in my case, with feno-fibrate (Tricor), pravastatin (Pravachol), and fish oil capsules and now just pravastatin—I have maintained normal blood lipid levels.

Another complication I experienced was contracting the Epstein-Barr virus. Although the level of the virus was high, I had no symptoms. Still, my doctors were concerned enough to call in a specialist on the virus to examine me. In his opinion, I required no specific treatment, but my doctors were instructed to monitor the virus carefully. Because they believed that the elevated level of the virus suggested that I was excessively immunosuppressed, they decided to lower my dose of tacrolimus.

Reducing the amount of immunosuppressants I was receiving could have placed my kidney at risk of rejection. However, lowering the dose of my medication not only reduced the level of the virus but also lowered my blood creatinine. If my body were rejecting my kidney, my blood creatinine would have risen. Because antire-jection drugs can damage the kidney, less immunosuppression actually helped in my case.

My experience with a clinical trial may not be typical. Being part of an experimental program to reduce the amount of immu-nosuppression needed, rather than getting a transplant under stan-dard care, probably reduced my risk of rejection owing to viral infections. A friend of mine died from complications of lymphoma resulting from a high degree of immunosuppression. In his case, he lost his kidney and passed away after a dialysis treatment. This was another reason why I chose to enroll in the clinical trial.

Six months after my transplant, I no longer had to take the antimicrobial medications and took only a low dose of tacrolimus as my immunosuppressant. At that point, I felt great and started creating my new life. To determine whether a clinical trial is right for you, consult your nephrologist for help.

I should emphasize that clinical trials are available for all sorts of diseases, including those that cause CKD. It would be valu-able for you to consider enrolling in one of them, if appropriate, depending on your medical and personal circumstances. Check www.clinicaltrials.gov for available studies.

As we learned earlier in the chapter, kidney transplantations have very high rates of success. Most of the transplant recipients whom I know personally, regardless of whether they received them through a standard protocol or a clinical trial, have responded very well to their new organs. Some had complications, but they eventually healed and are enjoying life to the fullest. So can you! If you have no significant complications after your transplant, you, too, can live a normal life, and CKD can become a distant memory.

CHAPTER 8

Future Treatment Options

THROUGHOUT THIS BOOK, I have discussed currently available treatments for people with chronic kidney disease (CKD). I have also discussed options for treating the causes of it. This chapter looks ahead to what the future may hold in terms of new treatments for people with failing kidneys. In addition, I shall review the advances in kidney disease research since the last edition of this book was published. Progress in some areas has been very encouraging.

In the 1950s, when my mother confronted CKD and kidney failure caused by polycystic kidney disease (PKD), there were no treatments for hypertension, anemia, or kidney failure. Neither dialysis nor transplantation was readily available for people with kidney failure from *any* cause. At the time, it was a death sentence.

Over the past five decades, however, dedicated research has yielded many new treatment options for people at risk for CKD. Not all of these new treatments are optimal, and their side effects sometimes impede quality of life. For example, although kidney transplantation is the treatment of choice for kidney failure, the availability of a donor kidney is uncertain, and the underlying disease might take its toll while the person is waiting for a transplant. In addition, once a transplant has been performed, the side effects of immunosuppressant drugs can be life threatening. If the prospect of CKD is in your future or in your children's future (that is, if your family has a strong genetic predisposition for CKD), looking ten to twenty years ahead at how the next generation might fare, may give you hope about the future of treatment. Although some of this discussion is speculative, the prospects are plausible. Only time will tell if any of these promising new approaches to treatment come to fruition.

New Therapeutic Approaches

The Human Genome Project, which sequenced the genes on each of the twenty-three human chromosomes (chapter 3), may allow scientists to find the proteins that each gene makes. With a comprehension of the role of these proteins in operating the biochemical reactions of our cells, we may begin to understand the underlying defects that cause disease. Substantial progress has been made over the past decade in understanding the underlying causes of CKD (chapter 3). As a result, research is under way to identify potential targets, such as receptors or enzymes involved in an abnormal response. Once the targets have been identified, researchers can develop new medications to work effectively with those targets.

Historically, developing a medication involves studying its overall effectiveness and safety in a *population* of people with a disease because not all people react to the drug in the same way. In study populations, responses vary, and researchers use analytical tools to decide whether a drug will be useful and safe in the clinic *on the average*. Because many genes could be involved with a disease, the response to a specific drug by a specific patient could be different from how the *average* person reacts to the drug; for example, the patient may react differently on the basis of the drug target or the way the patient's body processes the drug.[1]

Pharmacogenetics

In the future, doctors may be able to predict how an individual will respond to treatment, resulting in individualized health care tailor-made to a person's specific characteristics, not just to how people on average respond to a medication. Moreover, health care treatments may be modified based on a person's genetically mediated responses to a number of medications, some of which may be effective and some not. This new approach to treatment is called *pharmacogenetics.* Depending on the condition, this promising future treatment could analyze a person's genetic code to determine whether her genetic attributes support the use of a particular treatment.

Pharmacogenetics may also yield information about the target of the medication and how the body breaks down the drug. For example, the liver metabolizes drugs using enzymes, which have different activities, based on the variants of the genes involved. Identifying the genetic variants of a person's liver enzymes could help doctors prescribe drugs most likely to work according to that person's genetic makeup.

Although in its infancy, pharmacogenetics has already led to the development of better treatments for some diseases. It has been known since the 1950s that certain genetic variants in several enzymes that metabolize drugs in the liver can enhance or reduce their effectiveness. For example, identifying specific mutations in different cancers has helped tailor treatment with a drug that specifically works on that mutation. The treatment of hepatitis C had been greatly improved by the observation that a protein known as artificial interferon was more effective in patients with a particular genetic variant than in people without it. However, this treatment is no longer used because a combination of antiviral medications can now cure hepatic C infections.[2] In addition, this new treatment can cure infections in those receiving kidney transplants.

Whether a pharmacogenetic approach will yield improved treatments for kidney disease remains to be explored.[3] So far, no new treatments based on this approach have come to market. We still need a better understanding of the mechanisms underlying different kidney diseases, but the approach may be more valuable for treating some illnesses but not all. Because a specific disease can be associated with many variations in the genetic code, as is the case with diabetes, any specific variation might contribute a great deal—or very little—to the expression of the disease. Even then, a mutation and the actions of the protein made by the gene may not be significantly responsible for the clinical symptoms of a disease. Thus, pharmacogenetics holds the most promise with diseases with only a few genes contributing to the expression of the disease, such as PKD and, perhaps, some glomerular diseases, such as Alport's syndrome, IgA nephropathy, and FSGS (focal segmental glomerulosclerosis). Depending on how many genes are involved in these diseases and the number of altered biochemical pathways, multiple drugs with different mechanisms of action may be needed to effectively treat these diseases, a so called cocktail of medications.

Individualized treatment based on a person's genetic code is not a far-fetched idea. The cost of performing the sequencing has plummeted dramatically in recent years. Sequencing one person's complete genome costs under $1,000 and could be as little as $100 in the near future. Sequencing a child's entire genome at birth may become a routine procedure. Because a person's genome does not change over time, it would be necessary to sequence each person's genome only once, and therefore this would be a onetime expense. As we begin understanding how and when genes turn on and off, it may be possible to determine which genes are overactive or underactive in a disease state and then tailor the treatment to the process that a specific gene mediates. Currently, it is possible in diseases like cancer to predict the response to a particular form of treatment based on a certain genetic characteristic of the patient.

There is a downside to genome sequencing and to knowing a person's predispositions to specific diseases. For one thing, a predisposition to a disease does not necessarily mean a person will get the disease. Many diseases develop only when people who have the genes that make them susceptible to the disease encounter something in the environment, like a virus, which turns the disease "on." Some critics argue that genetic sequencing could cause people to worry needlessly, because they might never develop a disease, even though their genes indicate that they have the *potential* to develop the disease. There is also some concern that worried individuals will get unnecessary medical procedures to monitor for disease. Also, evidence that a person is at risk for a specific health condition might lead insurers or employers to discriminate against that person. To combat this concern in the United States, the Genetic Information Nondiscrimination Act was signed into law in 2008; this act specifically forbids such discrimination based on genetic information. In addition, the passage of the Patient Protection and Affordable Care Act in 2010 also prohibits this type of discrimination.

Drug Repurposing

In the history of medicine, thousands of drugs have been developed to treat a whole host of diseases. An exciting development in drug discovery has been how some of these drugs can effectively treat another condition not necessarily related to its original use. This new approach, called *drug repurposing*, could revolutionize the development of new treatments.[4] The main advantages of this approach are bypassing drug screening to find candidate drugs for clinical trials and early phase clinical trials to establish safety. This approach can save hundreds of millions of dollars in developmental costs. A few examples of drug repurposing are aspirin, a pain reliever, used as a blood thinner to reduce cardiac events; sildenafil (Viagra), a blood pressure reducer, used to treat erectile dysfunction; and thalidomide, a treatment for morning sickness, used to treat multiple myeloma.

Drug repurposing has been used in the treatment of kidney disease. The best example is tolvaptan (Jynarque) to treat PKD. It was originally used to treat those with low sodium blood levels. It worked by promoting urination without the loss of electrolytes by blocking the actions of vasopressin, a hormone that promotes fluid retention. Researchers found that inhibiting this mechanism reduced the growth of cysts, thereby reducing the loss of kidney function (chapters 3 and 5). Tolvaptan, approved by the Food and Drug Administration, is the first drug to treat PKD.

Another example of drug repurposing is a treatment for protecting kidneys from functional decline in people with diabetes. Usually, drugs that control blood sugar do not protect the kidneys. However, empagliflozin (Jardiance), canagliflozin (Invokana), and dapagliflozin (Farxiga) not only control blood sugar but also reduce the decline of kidney function. Although this example may not meet a strict definition of drug repurposing, it represents an action that was not originally studied. Whether these drugs might also treat kidney diseases from other causes awaits further research, but it looks promising (chapter 3).

Gene Editing

As discussed in chapter 3, genetic mutations cause many diseases. With their playing such a role, could using a technique to change our genes aid in finding treatments and cures? A new technique that can change the sequence of a strand of DNA or even replace one mutated letter makes it possible to do just that, the ability to do *gene editing*. This technique uses a tool called *CRISPR*, which stands for Clusters of Regularly Interspersed Short Palindromic Repeats, which allows researchers to cut out strands of mutated DNA and replace them with the correct sequence. CRISPR is also known as CRISPR-Cas9. The Cas9 is an enzyme that does the cutting. A DNA template of the correct sequence can then be inserted where the cut or cuts were made. The development of CRISPR led to the awarding of the 2020 Nobel Prize in Chemistry to Emmanuelle Charpentier and Jennifer Doudna for their pioneering work.

Researchers have made great strides in using CRISPR to correct human diseases, such as cystic fibrosis, cataracts, and Fanconi anemia (a disease that causes bone marrow failure and leads to various cancers).[5] CRISPR might also be useful in controlling insects that inflict disease, such as mosquitos that cause malaria. Could this technique be used to treat or cure the complex causes of kidney disease? Recent research suggests that it might.

Although CRISPR has not been used in humans to correct mutations involved with kidney diseases, it has proved important to researchers who model how changes in genetic sequences can affect disease in laboratory animals and cell systems.[6] A goal is showing that specific mutations have corresponding biochemical changes that then are responsible for the pathological changes seen in kidney diseases. Historically, this has been difficult to do in humans and even other live animals. It is important to know if a gene mutation is not only necessary but also sufficient to show that it is the underlying cause of a kidney disease, although ultimately, it may result from alterations in numerous biochemical pathways. The alterations would have to be linked to the pathology of the disease.

An interesting model recently developed involves forming *organoids* from stem cells that can form a structure in cell cultures with several working parts of a kidney, rather than just one cell type. This technique has been used to study PKD, FSGS, Alport's syndrome, and metabolic syndrome. If CRISPR could be used to modify genes in organoids, these techniques could lay the foundation for possibly altering genes in laboratory animals and eventually humans to cure genetic diseases.

The concept of *gene therapy* has many medical, ethical, and legal implications. Although curing an inherited disease might sound like the holy grail, it depends on getting everything right. One big issue is selectivity of the gene correction. CRISPR is not yet 100 percent capable of changing a gene without errors. A treatment may inadvertently induce mutations of its own through copying errors or changes in other genes that might have adverse effects on a patient. Newer gene editing techniques, such as *prime editing*, might avoid this problem in the future.[7] Prime editing can do a better job of precisely cutting DNA than traditional CRISPR does and has been successful in correcting mutations with fewer problems in sickle cell anemia and Tay-Sachs disease. With further advances in gene editing techniques, people may be cured successfully of all sorts of genetically based diseases.

To truly eradicate an inherited disease, gene editing of the germline cells would be needed. These are the cells that carry genetic information to the next generation, that is, sperm and eggs. Cloning various species and changing their genetic composition shows that this can be done. But, creating designer babies with specific, preplanned attributes in addition to or instead of curing an inherited disease is a major ethical and perhaps legal concern of gene editing. Deciding how or whether to proceed will require debate by medical professionals, ethicists, and legal leaders, with ultimate agreement of citizens, before gene editing is done in people. Although those of us who are affected with inherited kidney diseases would want a cure for ourselves and our children and grandchildren, it must be done carefully and with full knowledge of the ramifications of what we are doing.

Biological Markers

Diagnosis and treatment of kidney diseases are important in medicine. However, wouldn't it be valuable to detect accurately the very earliest signs or indicators that a disease has begun? Now, doctors use blood tests, such as creatinine to calculate GFR (glomerular filtration rate), and urine analysis to look for protein (albumin) to diagnose kidney disease once the damage is already done. In addition, they have clues that kidney function may be a risk factor by looking for family history of the disease or finding someone has high blood pressure or high blood glucose. These factors only suggest possible risk, not inevitability. If the very beginnings of kidney disease could be determined, perhaps earlier in life, better strategies could be developed to further reduce the decline in kidney function and better predict progression to kidney failure. In addition, being able to assess the effectiveness of a treatment would also be valuable. This is where good, predictive *biological markers* could be very beneficial.[8]

Research in the area of biomarkers of kidney disease is still in its early phase. Many markers have been proposed, but the one looking most promising for early diagnosis and prognosis is CKD273, a panel of 273 urinary proteins mostly involved with collagen. The value of CKD273 has been in predicting the decline in kidney function in people with diabetes.[9] The marker also correlates with the degree of scarring in the kidney. Many other proteins are being studied (too many to discuss here) but are still in the early stage of investigation. A big step forward would be finding which proteins are markers for the different kidney diseases, so that nephrologists could discriminate among the various diseases for a better diagnosis. The important takeaway is biological markers in kidney disease look very promising and will, hopefully, be used soon in a clinical setting to diagnose and treat kidney disease at very early stages.

Dialysis

People who have been on dialysis know that it is an often unpleasant treatment for kidney failure. Although dialysis keeps us alive and can improve our quality of life, it can be uncomfortable and has numerous other drawbacks. As we learned in chapter 6, both peritoneal dialysis and hemodialysis have their pros and cons.

Peritoneal dialysis allows us to perform our own treatment but can be inconvenient in terms of where we can perform exchanges. In addition, peritoneal dialysis causes weight gain and loss of protein and carries the risk of peritonitis. Hemodialysis must be performed on a specific schedule that may not be convenient, especially considering the demands of employment. People on hemodialysis may experience side effects such as lightheadedness, nausea, bleeding from the fistula or graft, and infections. To have hemodialysis, people must take a great deal of time out of their normal schedules to make clinical visits several times a week. Regardless of what form of dialysis we choose, the drawbacks can take a toll.

A big step forward over the past decade is the greater use and acceptance of home hemodialysis. With smaller dialysis machines, the setup requires less floor space than older, larger models did. Moreover, home dialysis can be performed more on a patient's schedule rather than on the dialysis facility's schedule. More frequent sessions at home can provide better outcomes, helping patients feel better.

A variation of this approach is nightly home hemodialysis, in which patients dialyze using a slower flow rate while they sleep, with a typical treatment lasting seven hours. Proponents of nightly home hemodialysis claim that patients maintain better control of their blood chemistries, have fewer problems with anemia, have better blood pressure control, and spend less time in the hospital.[10] The current number, organization, and location of technicians and nurses are not adequate to process the increased workload of daily, in-center treatments, even though this approach might benefit many patients. Thus, home hemodialysis can make more frequent sessions possible. A big advance for pursuing this path is Medicare and health insurance companies now routinely cover the costs of these techniques. A drawback to nightly home hemodialysis is that it can be difficult to secure the needles in the access to avoid serious and potentially life-threatening bleeding. Often, people on hemodialysis need a properly trained partner to assist in inserting needles and monitoring the session. Nonetheless, home hemodialysis is here to stay and provides another option for dialysis that was not routinely available even ten years ago.

Also under development are wearable hemodialysis machines to allow for more frequent dialysis.[11] These designs use small minipumps and dialyzers but have sorbent systems, which absorb the dialysate and clean and recirculate it, reducing the need for a large fluid source. The two machines under study are a wearable machine that can be carried strapped around your waist or in a backpack or implanted inside the body. All these approaches are designed to give dialysis patients more freedom of movement than standard forms of hemodialysis provide. Several small-scale human trials have been conducted to test the effectiveness of these devices, but larger ones are not yet ongoing, according to www.clinicaltrials .gov. Still in the early stages of development, wearable hemodialysis units have the potential to increase the quality of life of patients by improving their medical outcomes and reducing the amount of time they spend strapped to a dialysis machine. Given the slow start-up and progress, it may be many years before wearable hemo-dialysis machines will be practical.

Finally, artificial filters or dialyzers that are more efficient might improve the medical results of hemodialysis. Because the crux of hemodialysis is the dialyzer, improving its filtering capabilities, while sparing the integrity of red blood cells and reducing stress on the body, could improve medical outcomes for patients. As dis-cussed in chapter 6, some newer dialyzers are able to retain protein better, remove larger toxins, and remove excess phosphate. Per-haps, dialyzers of the future will be even more effective.

Transplantation

Receiving a kidney transplant is a great gift of life, whether you were on dialysis or were fortunate enough to get a new kidney before your kidneys completely failed, a preemptive transplant. The freedom that a transplant gives is immeasurable. Although you must take medications for the rest of the useful life of your kidney, it is far better than being tethered to a dialysis machine.

As we saw in chapter 7, the biggest risk associated with an organ transplant is rejection. Because the body perceives the new kidney as a foreign invader, the immune system will attempt to destroy it. Detecting rejection early would be important in the long-term viability of the transplant. Therefore, as part of the post-transplantation care regimen, transplant recipients take drugs that suppress the immune system. The immune-suppressing medications available today are quite good in preventing rejection. However, there are serious potential side effects. A suppressed immune system increases the risks of contracting infections and some forms of cancer. Some of these conditions can be life threatening. In addition, the risks of developing diabetes, cardiovascular disease, and osteoporosis increase.

A possible solution to these complications may be the development of immunosuppressants targeted to the part of the immune system responsible for rejection. Currently, physicians use medications that suppress *all* cell-mediated immune functions. In the future, new drugs might target immune functions that relate only to transplanted organs. That approach would put much less stress on the body.

Immune Tolerance

Another approach currently under study but not yet widely used is lowering the response of the immune system to the presence of a foreign organ, a process called *tolerance*.[12] I participated in such a study when I received my transplant (chapter 7). The premise involved depleting my body of the cells that cause rejection—T-cells—for about two weeks, which allowed enough time for my body to get used to the new kidney. As a result, I needed far less immunosuppression than is usually required, thereby reducing my risk of developing the complications that often result from the standard protocol. Sixteen years post-transplant, I have had no rejection episodes, although I take very little antirejection medication, compared to a recipient receiving standard care. Various other approaches have been taken to develop tolerance to a donor's kidney.[13] With further research, one or more of these approaches, using bone marrow transplants and stem cells from the donor, could be tailored to the individual patient. Eventually, it may be possible to avoid rejection altogether.

Xenotransplantation

With the lack of sufficient supply of kidneys for transplantation, one intriguing line of research, called *xenotransplantation*, involves assessing whether kidneys from animals (such as pigs, which have kidneys structurally similar to human kidneys) could be used as donors for human transplants. Although it would seem almost certain that the recipient's body would reject the kidney from another species, scientists have been genetically engineering pigs, so their kidneys are immunologically less reactive or inactive in a human patient. Another difficulty with xenotransplantation has been the risk that the animal's organs might contain retroviruses that could infect a recipient.

Some progress has been made to make pig kidneys more viable for human transplantation.[14] Over the past decade, survival times of pig kidneys transplanted into monkeys have increased from twenty-three days to ten months. This is due to better genetic engineering techniques to make the pig kidneys more like those of nonhuman primates. Similar genetic improvements could make pig kidneys less likely to provoke rejection in humans. Some advances in immunosuppressive drugs have reduced rejection even more. Perhaps, further manipulating the pig genome will eventually eliminate pig retroviruses as a problem.

So, when will we see pig kidneys transplanted into humans? Not anytime soon. Finding the right candidates even for a clinical trial may be difficult because of ethical concerns.[15] People might find the idea of having a pig organ repugnant, and it could disrupt their sense of self. In addition, religious reasons could be raised, especially among Jews and Muslims who view pigs as unclean. However, attitudes can change under the right conditions. The FDA suggests that xenotransplantation be reserved for those who do not have other viable treatment options for life-threatening conditions and would significantly benefit from improving their quality of life. Over the next decade, we will see how this potential transplant option progresses, and if it is a viable and practical one.

Stem Cells

Stem cells may prove to be another promising avenue of increasing options for transplantations. Shortly after fertilization of an egg, when cells begin dividing, these cells are *undifferentiated*, that is, they are not kidney, brain, skin, heart, or bone cells. The cells at that stage are considered *pluripotent*. With further development of the embryo, pluripotent stem cells can be transformed or *differentiated* into the various cells of the body used to make organs. Under the proper conditions, pluripotent stem cells someday may be used to grow new body parts, including kidneys, for people who need them.

Pluripotent stem cells can come from either embryonic cells (from human embryos or human umbilical cord blood) or adult cells transformed into pluripotent stem cells. Although researchers are studying pluripotent stem cells as precursors for making specialized cells to correct many diseases, the moral implications of using embryonic stem cells have hampered research for this purpose. Nevertheless, several approaches using pluripotent stem cells have been explored over the last decade to obtain proof of concept.

When kidneys fail, only two treatments are available: dialysis or transplantation. Previously, it has been thought that damaged kidneys could not be fixed. It would be great if that was not true! Researchers have been exploring just such a treatment. The aim is to use pluripotent stem cells to rejuvenate and restore kidney function. Two lines of research are unfolding: restore kidney function in the existing diseased kidney and build a new one from a patient's cells.

Studies using different types of stem cells and animal models have shown some success in improving kidney function in rodents, but not in larger animals.[16] It is not clear why this approach has not worked in these animals, but at some point, I expect this problem will be solved. Although stem-cell kidney regeneration looks promising, it may take a while to find the right cell types to use and a consistent protocol before this approach can find its way into the clinic.

With the availability of kidneys for transplantation still scarce, other sources of kidneys would be desirable. If you have a damaged kidney, why not make a new one? What would you need to build one, especially with so many specialized cells required for it to function and with a way to hold them together as a viable organ? This is not as far-fetched as it may sound. Over the past decade, several laboratories have used stem cells to create kidney-like structures of increasing complexity. These attempts have succeeded to initially produce a single-cell type of the kidney up to the development of organoids, discussed earlier, with several cell types that can self-organize.[17] Organoids appear to be an intermediate stage in the development of a transplantable kidney. However, several big hurdles remain, including getting a blood supply to the group of cells, having a way to remove urine, and having a structure on which to make a fully functional, lab-grown kidney.

A new approach that might solve some if not all these problems is the *organoid-on-a-chip*.[18] Unlike regular organoids that get their nutrients by diffusion from the surrounding environment that ultimately restricts their growth, organoids can be placed in extremely small chambers in which the environment can be controlled to simulate an organ outside a living being. Using this technique, kidney organoids could grow blood vessels and more mature cells than the organoids would do on their own, resembling kidney formation in the embryo.[19]

Finally, what might facilitate the development of a structure on which cells could adhere and grow is the introduction of *3D printing* into the process.[20] 3D printing deposits one or more chosen materials one layer at a time, according to a computerized design. The trick is finding a surface template that will allow cells to adhere to it, thrive, and form a functional organ.[21] Progress continues with better materials being developed for a scaffold. Getting to a functional kidney is a long way off, but the use of 3D printing may help eventually in providing a solution to the shortage of kidneys for those in need.

Whether any of these approaches to addressing the kidney shortage for transplantation will work will take decades of further research. If one or a combination of them work, there is still the issue of using embryonic stem cells to produce organs. It is not likely that the moral issue will be resolved to the point that society would find their use acceptable. The ultimate solution is using adult stem cells from a patient and making them into a new kidney. Putting cost, time, and other hurdles aside, here is a scenario that might be acceptable.

Since adult stem cells can be converted to pluripotent stem cells, imagine taking a skin sample from a patient and converting these cells through a series of steps to pluripotent stem cells. From these cells, transform them into kidney cells and grow them outside the body to form a transplantable kidney. This might be done with some of the techniques described above or newer more advanced ones. Once implanted, the patient would not need immunosuppressive drugs because the original material came from the patient. This approach should have no ethical problems associated with using embryonic stem cells.

Based on current state-of-the-art science, the scenario that I have described seems impossible, but advances occur all the time and often rapidly. A big problem is not knowing enough about the complex process the body uses to create an organ from stem cells. During fetal development, various genes turn on and off at various times to construct each organ. However, the advent of organoids and organoids-on-a-chip gives us an inkling of what is possible and how this process works.

FROM THE VARIOUS possible options for improving treatment described in this chapter, which of them are most likely to develop into viable treatments over the next decade? As I look into my crystal ball, reducing the progression of CKD with new drugs, some of them repurposed, looks most likely. Genetic approaches for treatment, xenotransplantation, and making new kidneys must overcome many obstacles to potentially be useful options for nephrologists to treat their patients.

Scientists are pursuing different avenues of research at the same time. Anyone who reads the newspaper or listens to radio or watches television knows that breakthroughs in medical treatment happen all the time. We should expect such developments in kidney disease research. One day another edition of this book will be needed, because the causes and treatments of CKD will have advanced so far that current treatments will be outdated.

I look forward to writing that new edition.

Epilogue

IT CAN BE DEVASTATING to receive a diagnosis of failing kidneys. It can be daunting to anticipate what lies ahead, including the difficulties of treatment. Educating yourself about the decisions you must make, as well as using all the tools available to you, will help you manage the process. Ultimately, it will be up to you to decide how hard chronic kidney disease (CKD) will be for you.

Throughout this book, I have emphasized the importance of taking responsibility for your health. Accepting that you are primarily responsible for your health will empower you as you face the prospect of CKD.

You now have a great deal of information about how to prevent or postpone CKD. It is time to start implementing what you know. For some of you, the problem may seem far in the future and perhaps secondary to the other priorities of life that compete for your attention. However, this is no time to be in denial. No priority is more important than your life. Without your health, nothing else will matter. I learned that lesson when my kidneys were failing. You have a choice: take action now and prevent or postpone the problem or suffer the consequences of inaction in the future.

Take control of your health. No one should be more motivated than you are to improve your future quality of life. Your family and friends can help you, but understand that they have only so much time and energy to lend. Find ways to help yourself and do not depend totally on others, not even your doctors. Your doctors may give their best medical advice, but they are not responsible for implementing their advice. *You are!* Use the advice in this book and find ideas of your own that help you with your daily activities.

I know firsthand how tough it can be to take care of yourself when you are sick. With little energy, I had great difficulty even getting up in the morning, let alone taking care of routine, daily tasks. But on many days, you will be well enough to do at least some of the most important things that require your attention. We all make occasional bad decisions or feel overwhelmed about our health situation. Try not to dwell on the setbacks. Celebrate your accomplishments and push aside your failures.

CKD is a serious condition. But with commitment, patience, and practice you can make it. Along the way, create the life you want.

Remember:

Move quickly through denial and face your disease directly.

Be your own advocate.

Believe your life will improve.

Take the long view.

Remain optimistic and give a positive spin to everything.

Know your priorities and stick to them.

Be willing to take risks.

Ask for help, but don't depend on it.

Keep your sense of humor.

Appendix

Chronic kidney disease (CKD) and especially kidney failure have been increasing rapidly worldwide over the past two decades, affecting almost one billion people and killing nearly one million, based on 2013 data.[1] Mostly, CKD is caused by diabetes, hypertension, and advancing age and touches the lives of men more than women. Here is some insight into what the world has experienced.

The number of people with CKD (called *prevalence*) is not uniform throughout the world, and deaths from kidney failure are often higher in countries without enough facilities or financial resources for dialysis and transplantation. In other cases, significant minority populations are present that tend to have higher prevalence rates of CKD than the majority population has. Examples of the latter case are the United States, Canada, and Australia, whose minority populations show prevalence rates two to ten times higher than the majority population.

Regions of the world differ in their rates of kidney failure, averaging 1,200 cases per million population.[2] In 2016, the highest prevalence rates of kidney failure were in Taiwan (3,392), Japan (2,599), and the United States (2,196) and lowest in Bangladesh (117), South Africa (181), and Ukraine (188). The number of new cases (called *incidence*) was highest in Taiwan (493), the United States (378), and the Jalisco region of Mexico (355) and lowest in South Africa (21), Ukraine (32), and Belarus (51).

If we look at various regions of the world, prevalence and incident rates can be quite different within the region. In the Americas, the United States (2,196) and Canada (1,346) had the highest on average for 2016[2,3] and incidence rates of 378 per million and 200 per million, respectively. On the other hand, Latin America had the lowest prevalence, based on 2010 data, averaging 660 per million.[4] Of the nations and territories studied, Puerto Rico (1,355),

Chile (1,137), Uruguay (1,031), and Mexico (975) had the highest rates, whereas Nicaragua (37), Paraguay (149), Bolivia (153), and the Dominican Republic (165) had the lowest rates. Incidence rates were highest in Mexico (458) and Puerto Rico (369) and lowest in Guatemala (11), Paraguay (33), and Peru (34).

In Europe, prevalence rates of kidney failure vary widely as well.[2,5] The overall rate was 828 per million in 2016. In the countries for which data were available, Portugal (1,906), France (1,278), and Spain (1,234), had the highest rates, whereas Ukraine (188), Belarus (289), Russia (310), and Albania (507) had the lowest rates. In the United Kingdom, the prevalence was 956 per million. Incidence rates of kidney disease, with an average of 121 per million, were highest in Greece (251), the Czech Republic (243), and Portugal (236), whereas Ukraine (29), Russia (59), and Belarus (62) had the lowest rates. In the United Kingdom, the incidence was 116 per million.

Studies of kidney disease in Africa have varied in quality and are, therefore, difficult to put into context with the rest of the world.[6] Of those data considered medium to high quality, though, prevalence of CKD (rates for kidney failure were not available) ranged from 2 to 41 percent, with a pooled estimate of 10.8 percent. Estimates suggest that CKD was highest in West Africa (16.5%) and lowest in North Africa (4%). The remainder of Africa had estimated rates intermediate between the two extremes.

Of the countries surveyed in Asia, prevalence of kidney failure was highest in East Asia, such as Taiwan (3,392), Japan (2,599), Singapore (2,076), and South Korea (1,816) and lowest in South Asia in Bangladesh (117) and Indonesia (323).[2] Incidence mirrored the prevalence, in that the same countries had the highest incidence, ranging from 493 per million in Taiwan to 259 per million in Malaysia.

Prevalence and incidence were lower in the Middle East than those in East Asia, with Saudi Arabia (826 and 145, respectively) and Kuwait (787 and 141, respectively) being highest in the region and lowest in Iraq (251, prevalence) and Iran (81, incidence). However, the prevalence of diabetes was high, suggesting that kidney disease is likely to increase in the Middle East in the future.[7,8] Interestingly, the two most populated countries in Asia, India and China, do not have well-characterized statistics. However, since the number of people with diabetes is expanding in both countries, the risk for kidney disease is also expected to rise in the coming years.[9,10]

Finally, Australia and New Zealand have a significant minority of Indigenous people whose high prevalence and incidence can be lost when looking at the whole population. In Australia and New Zealand, the prevalence of kidney disease was 988 per million and 966 per million, respectively, in 2016, whereas the incidence was 120 per million and 122 per million.[2,11] However, in the Indigenous populations those numbers were five to nine times higher and, in this case, affected women more than men.[11,12]

In summary, CKD leading to kidney failure is a major problem, though not uniformly, throughout the world. The United States, Canada, East Asia, and Western Europe have the greatest problems with kidney failure, whereas much of Latin America, South Asia, and Eastern Europe have the least problems. The major cause is diabetes. Kidney failure is seen more often in men than in women with only a few exceptions in minority populations. Although some regions of the world have a higher problem with kidney failure than others do, the reasons for this are not yet understood, although it may have to do with diet (chapter 5).

Resources

This resource list is for readers interested in learning more about kidney diseases, how the kidney functions, the diagnosis and management of kidney diseases, the principles of dialysis and kidney transplantation, and other topics not covered in detail in this book. Readers who wish to get involved in a community of patients and health care providers can use the list to identify and contact organizations whose sole purpose is to support patients. Some of these organizations advocate for patients and include congressional lobbying as part of their activities on behalf of patients.

The list of resources and organizations is not exhaustive but does include sources that I found most informative and authoritative.

Educational Resources

The internet is a seemingly unlimited source of information. Websites provide information and support, and scientific databases link to primary research articles on kidney diseases. The National Library of Medicine at the National Institutes of Health provides the best databases (see www.nlm.nih.gov). The most useful database for the public is PubMed. PubMed is easy to use for simple searches; begin your searches at www.pubmed.gov. In addition, the website of the National Institute of Diabetes and Digestive and Kidney Diseases has a great deal of information on kidney disease that is easy to read (see www.niddk.nih.gov/health-information /kidney-disease), but not necessarily current.

Several of these organizations exist for the sole purpose of supporting kidney patients in general and those with specific diseases. Here are some of them:

National Kidney Foundation
30 East 33rd Street
New York, NY 10016
Phone: 800-622-9010
Email: info@kidney.org
Website: www.kidney.org

The National Kidney Foundation (NKF) is an organization that provides exceptionally valuable information on kidney diseases in general, as well as on dialysis and transplantation. The NKF offers numerous pamphlets describing many different aspects of kidney failure. This is a useful site for learning basic information about kidney failure. Recently, they established a program with the Fresenius Medical Care Foundation to help patients find donors for transplantation.

American Association of Kidney Patients
14440 Bruce B. Downs Blvd.
Tampa, FL 33613
Phone: 800-749-2257
Email: info@aakp.org
Website: www.aakp.org

The American Association of Kidney Patients has a site devoted to patient issues. According to their website, the organization "exists to serve the needs, interests, and welfare of all kidney patients and their families. Its mission is to improve the lives of fellow kidney patients and their families by helping them to deal with the physical, emotional, and social impact of kidney disease." The website has extensive information on all aspects of kidney disease.

American Diabetes Association
2451 Crystal Drive, Suite 900
Alexandria, VA 22202
Phone: 800-DIABETES (800-342-2383)
Website: www.diabetes.org

According to their website, the main mission of the American Diabetes Association is "to prevent and cure diabetes and to improve the lives of all people affected by diabetes." The site has extensive information for patients and professionals about diabetes, management of the disease, preventative measures, weight loss, and statistics. The American Diabetes Association also provides grants to help support research on diabetes.

American Heart Association
National Center
7272 Greenville Avenue
Dallas, TX 75231
Phone: 800-242-8721
Email: Through the website
Website: www.americanheart.org

The website of the American Heart Association provides information on many aspects of cardiovascular disease, including hypertension. One division of the American Heart Association is the American Stroke Association, which provides information on warning signs, prevention, and care for stroke patients.

American Stroke Association
National Center
7272 Greenville Avenue
Dallas, TX 75231
Phone: 888-478-7653
Email: Through the website
Website: www.strokeassociation.org

No organization is devoted specifically to glomerulonephritis. The website www.mayoclinic.com provides good information on the disease. In addition, two organizations exist specifically to address two causes of glomerulonephritis: the Alport Syndrome Foundation and IgA Nephropathy Support Network.

Alport Syndrome Foundation
PO Box 4130
Scottsdale, AZ 85261-4130
Phone: 480-800-3510
Website: www.alportsyndrome.org

Alport's syndrome is a genetic kidney disease. The mission of the Alport Syndrome Foundation is "to improve the lives of those affected by Alport syndrome through education, empowerment, advocacy and research. Our vision is to conquer Alport syndrome."

IgA Nephropathy Support Network
89 Ashfield Road
Shelburne Falls, MA 01370
Phone: 413-625-9339
Website: www.igansupport.org

The mission of the IgA Nephropathy Support Network is "to assist patients with IgA nephropathy and their families; to serve as a clearinghouse for dissemination of information about IgA nephropathy; and to promote research for a possible cure." The network provides newsletters and pamphlets.

PKD Foundation
1001 East 101st Terrace, Suite 220
Kansas City, MO 64131
Phone: 800-PKD-CURE
Email: pkdcure@pkdcure.org
Website: www.pkdcure.org

The best place to obtain useful and reliable information on polycystic kidney disease (PKD) is through the PKD Foundation, which
provides educational material for people with PKD, their families, and other interested parties. In addition, it funds grants to
researchers who are working to identify the causes of PKD as well
as potential treatments and cures for this inherited kidney disease.
The PKD Foundation is the only organization in the world that
addresses PKD exclusively. I did not discuss autosomal recessive
PKD (ARPKD) in this book because most patients have autosomal
dominant PKD (ADPKD). For readers interested in ARPKD, a place
to start learning more is found at the link on the PKD Foundation
website.

Nutrition

As we learned in chapter 5, it can be difficult for a person with
kidney disease to eat a proper diet and maintain good nutrition,
because of a limited list of permitted foods. This is especially true
for anyone on hemodialysis. The American Association of Kidney
Patients publishes a useful brochure that lists the sodium, potassium, protein, and caloric content of a wide variety of foods.
This brochure can help you in selecting meals that meet the requirements of hemodialysis. You can download it from https://
aakp.org/wp-content/uploads/woocommerce_uploads/2016/10
/Nutrition-Counter.pdf.

People on dialysis, especially peritoneal dialysis, generally must
have protein supplementation. Liquid supplements designed for dialysis patients are available, but they are expensive. For me, a better

alternative was a protein powder derived from egg whites. You can purchase powdered egg whites at www.optimumnutrition.com or at a local GNC. The latter source is often cheaper. Amazon.com also sells a selection of egg-white protein powder. See if they have cheaper options. Buying in five-pound containers is the least expensive option by volume. Note: *do not buy whey protein*. Whey protein, derived from dairy products, has a high phosphorus content.

Transplant Donor Websites

Because there is a shortage of kidneys available for transplantation, efforts are under way to identify more living donors. Several organizations have become increasingly active in matching living donors.

Alliance for Paired Donation
PO Box 965
Perrysburg, OH 43552
Phone: 419-360-7445
Email: admin@paireddonation.org
Website: www.paireddonation.org

Through a nationwide computer-matching program, the Alliance for Paired Donation helps arrange for living donations between pairs of potential donors not compatible with the patients with whom they originally intended to donate (chapter 7). The organization has been in existence since 2000 and has arranged paired or chained donations using a special matching algorithm. Registration is easy and free.

National Kidney Registry
PO Box 460
Babylon, NY 11702-0460
Phone: 800-936-1627
Email: administration@kidneyregistry.org
Website: www.kidneyregistry.org

The National Kidney Registry was founded "to save and improve the lives of people facing kidney failure by increasing the quality, speed, and number of living donor transplants in the world as well as protecting living donors." Since its inception in 2007, it has facilitated over four thousand transplants. The cost is free for donors and recipients who work through one of the participating centers. Recently, they began reimbursing kidney donors in the paired exchange program for lost wages while recovering from surgery.

MatchingDonors.com, Inc.
766 Turnpike Street
Canton, MA 02021
Phone: 781-821-2204
Email: contactus@matchingdonors.com
Website: www.matchingdonors.com

According to its website, the organization was "created to give people in need of transplant surgery an active way to search for a live organ donor. Our goal is to increase the number of transplant surgeries and improve awareness of live organ donation." MatchingDonors .com, Inc. attempts to match prospective living donors with those in need of a transplant. As of May 2020, almost sixteen thousand people willing to donate kidneys have been listed. Patients pay a fee to be listed on the site. The amount depends on the length of the listing. It ranges from $49 for a seven-day trial membership to $595 for a lifetime membership. Currently, Medicare and insurance companies do not reimburse this expense. For those who cannot afford the fee, Matching Donors claims that it waives it.

Kidneybuzz.com
21520 Yorba Linda Blvd., Suite G238
Yorba Linda, CA 92887
Phone: 949-715-8788
Email: Through the website
Website: www.kidney.com/find-a-kidney-donor-program

Kidneybuzz.com has developed a Find A Kidney Donor Program to find patients a kidney donor. According to their website, space is limited. Although the cost of listing is $56 a month, no evidence of success has been presented.

IF YOU PURSUE living donations through any of these websites, you must do so in close consultation with your transplant team. It is not clear from the sites whether those involved in the organization adequately screen potential donors for possible medical conflicts or other disqualifying factors.

Financial Aid

The costs for dialysis and kidney transplantation are substantial. Although some private insurance provides coverage, not all insurance does, and many patients have no private insurance at all. A major source of funding for dialysis and transplantation comes from the federal government through Medicare and Medicaid. Medicare can provide significant assistance to those in need who meet eligibility requirements. Useful information can be found in the brochure *Medicare Coverage of Kidney Dialysis and Kidney Transplant Services* available at the Medicare website at www.medicare.gov/Publica tions/#results&keyword=kidney%20dialysis. For further information, you can call Medicare at 800-MEDICARE (800-486-4028). For Medicaid, a joint federal and state program, benefits vary depending on the state and eligibility requirements. Check with your state agency for further information. Starting in 2018, Medicare has begun paying for diabetes prevention programs.

The American Kidney Fund provides funds to defray expenses associated with dialysis and transplantation that insurance does not cover, as well as help subsidize health insurance premiums. The fund also provides disaster relief for those who have medications, renal diet foods, and clothing lost in natural disasters. Finally, they offer brochures about kidney function and kidney diseases and educational seminars.

American Kidney Fund
11921 Rockville Pike, Suite 300
Rockville, MD 20852
Phone: 800-638-8299
Email: www.helpline@kidneyfund.org
Home page: www.kidneyfund.org

Finally, county services provided by local governments or private organizations also assist in covering dialysis costs for transportation and transplantation. Check with the social worker at your dialysis or transplant center for guidance.

Smartphone Apps for Chronic Kidney Disease

In the age of technology and smartphones that can do things we only dreamed about just ten years ago, many aspects of our lives, including our health, can be tracked. With so many aspects of dealing with chronic kidney disease, can smartphone apps help keep track of it all? Already, many apps exist for patients to use that might help them. Of course, which apps to use depend in part on the platform on which they run: Android or Apple (iOS). Some run on both platforms; others do not. How do you choose the right one? A recent study tried to provide some answers.[1]

Of the many apps available, twelve Android only, eleven iOS only, and five dual-platform apps were identified for further testing. When evaluated by patients, nephrologists, and general consumers, the different groups did not agree on their usefulness.

Evidently, each group rated the apps on different criteria. However, seven apps got high marks from both patients and nephrologists. Here is a list of apps, platforms, and features:

CAPD Helper	Android	• Tracking blood pressure • Tracking weight over time • List of general medications • List of dialysis-related medications
Kidney Disease Assistant	iOS	• Tracking creatinine or GFR • Tracking proteinuria • Tracking blood pressure
My Kidneys, My Health Handbook	Both	• Education about CKD • Education about hypertension • Education about diabetes • Sharing information
Our Journey with Peritoneal Dialysis	Both	• Education about peritoneal dialysis
Record Weight for Dialysis Patients	iOS	• Tracking and summarizing weight
Syck	iOS	• Education about kidney transplant • Connecting patients with other ones
Transplant Hero–Medication Reminder	Both	• Keeping list of transplant medications • Reminding patients to take medications

What is apparent from this list is none of them does everything for CKD patients. Perhaps, that is asking too much. You may find use in the ones listed. Give them a try. I suspect, however, that you may not find one that exactly works for your needs. Perhaps, you don't want to use several of them. The future of apps for CKD patients may come from smartwatches (wearables). Smartwatches can monitor heart rate, general activity, foods you consume, and calories you burn. As the technology improves, measurements of blood pressure and blood glucose levels will be practical. Perhaps, a solution to developing the best app may come from a joint venture between a kidney-based organization, such as the National Kidney Foundation or the American Society of Nephrology, and a medical app developer. This approach may find the best solution for patients' needs.

Glossary

Acidosis. Buildup of acid in the blood.

Adrenal glands. Small organs sitting atop the kidneys that secrete aldosterone, promoting fluid and salt retention.

Albuminuria. Protein in the urine. Protein in the urine is a symptom of kidney disease.

Aldosterone. *See* adrenal glands.

Alport's syndrome. An inherited glomerular disease that not only affects the kidney but also vision and hearing.

Anemia. Low red blood cell count.

Aneurysm. Ballooning of a major blood vessel that can rupture, causing massive bleeding.

Angiotensin system. Regulates blood pressure when salt concentration is low; renin stimulates the conversion of angiotensin I to angiotensin II, which constricts blood vessels to raise blood pressure.

Antibody. A protein created be the immune system to attack and destroy foreign entities like microorganisms and organs transplanted from other people.

Antigen. "Name tag" on cells that identifies the cells as belonging to a specific individual.

Atherosclerosis. Buildup of plaque in blood vessels that can contribute to hypertension.

Autosomal dominant polycystic kidney disease (ADPKD). Dominant form of PKD; a child has a 50 percent chance of inheriting the disease from an affected parent.

Autosomal recessive polycystic kidney disease (ARPKD). Recessive form of PKD; a child has a 25 percent chance of inheriting the disease if both parents are carriers of the mutated gene, but the parents do not have ARPKD themselves.

Bariatric surgery. A procedure that reduces the size of the stomach, so that obese people can lose weight.

Beta cells. Those cells in the pancreas that produce insulin. The lack of insulin production or insulin resistance leads to diabetes.

Biological marker. A test that can find a disease before symptoms occur.

Biopsy. A procedure in which a small amount of tissue is removed from the body for investigation and testing.

Blood typing. The means for determining one person's blood type compatibility with another person's blood type. Compatible blood typing is usually needed for kidney transplantation.

Blood urea nitrogen (BUN). A measure of kidney function. A high value indicates declining kidney function.

Bone marrow. Soft tissue in bone that makes red blood cells.

Calcidiol. An intermediate form of vitamin D in the production of calcitriol.

Calcitriol. The most active form of vitamin D that the body uses. It does not require activation by the kidney and is often given to dialysis patients who cannot make their own calcitriol.

Calcium. An important mineral in keeping bones strong and a mediator in many biochemical pathways.

Carbohydrates. A group of sugars and starches that are a source of energy for the body.

Carbon dioxide. The main substance in exhaled breath. In the form of bicarbonate, it neutralizes acidity in the blood.

Catheter. Access to a major vein. Catheters are used primarily for dialysis but can be a means of administering medications or nourishment. They can also be used to drain urine from the bladder.

Cholecalciferol. The form of vitamin D typically found in supplements. Cholecalciferol does not have to be activated in the skin. *See* vitamin D.

Chromosome. Structure within the nucleus of the cell that houses the genetic code. Each cell in humans contains twenty-three pairs.

Chronic kidney disease (CKD). A condition in which elimination of wastes from the body slowly declines until it no longer effectively takes place.

Conservative care. Treatment given to patients who decline dialysis or transplantation. Involves making patients comfortable by treating symptoms, such as swelling, pain, nausea, and difficulties in breathing.

Continuous ambulatory peritoneal dialysis (CAPD). Requires four to five manual exchanges of abdominal fluid per day.

Continuous cyclic peritoneal dialysis (CCPD). Uses a machine (cycler) to perform exchanges during the night; some manual exchanges needed during the day.

Creatinine. A measure of kidney function. Creatinine is completely filtered by the kidney, making it a more accurate measure than BUN. A high value indicates declining kidney function.

Creatinine clearance. The amount of creatinine filtered by the kidney and passed into the urine. This is the most accurate measure of kidney function.

CRISPR. A technique used to edit a sequence of DNA in a gene to function in a different way. Used to find treatments for diseases that are inherited or caused by noninherited mutations.

Crossmatch. The last test performed to avert rejection of a donated kidney. A negative test result allows the transplantation to proceed.

Deoxyribonucleic acid (DNA). Blueprints for life; composed of long strings of nucleotide sequences containing the instructions for making up to three proteins.

Diabetic nephropathy. Diabetes-induced kidney failure.

Dialysate. The solution drained from the abdomen during a peritoneal dialysis exchange; also, the solution bathing a dialyzer in a hemodialysis machine.

Dialysis. A method of cleansing the blood of waste products.

Dialyzer. A filter containing tiny filaments bathed with dialysate; blood passes through the filaments and toxins diffuse into the dialysate.

Drug repurposing. Taking a drug that treats one ailment by using it to treat another.

Edema. Accumulation of fluid in soft tissues of the body, especially in the legs and ankles.

Electrolytes. Salts, such as sodium and potassium, which control many functions in the body.

Erythrocytes. Red blood cells, which carry oxygen throughout the body.

Erythropoietin (EPO). A hormone made by the kidney to stimulate production of red blood cells (erythrocytes).

Exchange. The process in peritoneal dialysis by which the dialysate is replaced.

Fistula. A vascular access created by joining an artery and a vein in an arm or leg, used for hemodialysis.

Focal segmental glomerulosclerosis (FSGS). A glomerular disease often seen in African Americans because of a genetic mutation in the apolipoprotein L1 (*APLO1*).

Gene editing. The ability to change sequences in DNA of a particular gene or genes to change their function. It is being tested to treat inherited diseases in which sequences of DNA are altered.

Genes. The instructions for making and running a cell; composed of sequences of DNA.

Gene therapy. A method of treating a disease by altering selected genes in the body.

Genetic testing. Used to determine whether someone has a specific disease, such as polycystic kidney disease.

Glomerular filtration rate (GFR). A measurement similar to creatinine clearance, but GFR is calculated from blood creatinine and takes into account age and race.

Glomerulus. A structure in the kidney that filters blood of its waste products.

Glucose. The main source of energy in the body.

Good Samaritan kidney donor. An anonymous person willing to donate a kidney to a pool of potential recipients who may never know who their donor was.

Gout. An inflammatory, arthritic disorder resulting from a buildup of blood uric acid.

Graft. A vascular access created by joining an artery and vein to each end of a Gore-Tex tube, used for hemodialysis.

Hematocrit. The volume of blood comprising red blood cells.

Hemodialysis. Filtration of the blood with a machine that circulates blood through a dialyzer.

Hemoglobin. A protein in red blood cells that carries oxygen through the body. Hemoglobin levels can drop as kidneys fail.

Heparin. A blood thinner used in hemodialysis to avoid clotting in the tubing and dialyzer.

HLA typing. The means for determining one person's cells' immune compatibility with another person's cells. This typing is used for matching donors to recipients for a kidney transplant.

Homeostasis. The process of keeping conditions in the body within a normal range.

Hormones. Substances, such as aldosterone and leptin, acting on receptors that change physiological function.

Hyperlipidemia. Elevated blood fats like cholesterol, saturated fats, and triglycerides.

Hypertension. Blood pressure above 140/90.

Immune tolerance. Occurs when the immune system has a decreased ability to identify and attack an invading organism or transplanted organ.

Immunoglobulin A nephropathy (IgA). A glomerular disease resulting from attacks of the body's antibodies on the glomerulus.

Incidence. The number of new cases of a disease.

Insulin. A pancreatic protein that regulates glucose levels in the blood by helping it pass into cells.

Insulin pump. An artificial pancreas that regulates the amount of insulin in the blood.

Insulin resistance. Reduced ability of insulin to enter cells, even when blood insulin levels are high.

Kidney failure. When the kidney no longer adequately eliminates wastes. At this point, dialysis or transplantation is needed for survival.

Kt/V. A measure of efficiency in hemodialysis.

Leptin. A hormone that regulates hunger by reducing appetite; may play a role in type 2 diabetes.

Lupus nephritis. A glomerular disease caused by systemic lupus erythematosus, a complex autoimmune disease that affects several organs of the body, including the kidney.

Lymphocytes. Cells within the immune system that protect the body from foreign organisms. T-lymphocytes attack transplanted organs, causing rejection.

Metabolites. Substances formed through a series of biochemical reactions. For example, proteins are broken down into urea.

Microbiome. Bacteria in the intestines.

Mutations. Mistakes made in copying genes that can cause a malfunction in the cellular processes and can lead to a disease like PKD.

Natriuretic peptides. Hormones that play a role in salt-sensitive high blood pressure.

Nephron. The basic unit of the kidney, composed of a glomerulus, tubules, and collecting ducts.

Nephrotic syndrome. Another term for glomerular disease that leads to scarring of the glomerulus.

Non-steroidal anti-inflammatory drugs (NSAIDS). A class of drugs, such as aspirin and ibuprofen, used to relieve pain but must be used carefully or avoided in those with kidney disease.

Osteoporosis. A condition where excess amounts of calcium are removed from bones, making them brittle and more easily fractured.

Paired kidney donation. A system that allows recipients of kidney transplants to swap donors when they are not compatible.

Pancreatic islet cells. Cells in the pancreas that make insulin.

Panel reactive antibody (PRA). A test to measure the number of antibodies in the blood to assess the likelihood of kidney rejection. The higher the value, the greater the potential for rejection.

Parathyroid hormone. A hormone secreted from the two parathyroid glands in the neck that promotes removal of calcium in bone into the blood. This action can lead to osteoporosis.

Peritoneal dialysis. Filtration of the blood with a solution in the abdomen.

Peritoneal equilibrium test (PET). A method to determine the adequacy of peritoneal dialysis by measuring the creatinine and urea in four hourly samples.

Peritonitis. Inflammation of the lining of the abdomen.

Pharmacogenetics. The use of genetic information to develop new medications. Specific mutations in genes and accompanied altered protein sequences of proteins can suggest mechanisms underlying a disease that can be potential targets for therapeutic intervention.

Phosphorus. An important substance in the generation of energy. Phosphorus accumulates in hemodialysis patients and can combine with calcium in the blood to form plaques in organs, possibly leading to organ failure.

Polycystic kidney disease (PKD). An inherited disease characterized by cysts that grow and ultimately destroy kidney function.

Polygenic diseases. Diseases caused by mutations in multiple genes.

Potassium. A salt that helps regulate heartbeat and brain function. High blood potassium levels can lead to heart block. Usually, high potassium can be treated by altering diet or prescribing medications.

Prevalence. The total number of people with a disease at a given time.

Proteins. Long chains of amino acids that operate cells and provide structure for the body.

Proteinuria. Protein in the urine. *See* albuminuria.

Receptors. Entities on or within cells that translate a signal from a hormone or drug into a physiological response; specific for certain chemical structures like a key fitting a lock.

Renal cysts. Fluid-filled sacs that grow in the kidney in those with polycystic kidney disease.

Renin. A substance released from the kidney that activates the angiotensin system (*see* angiotensin system). Under normal circumstances, it helps maintain blood pressure during dehydration or extreme blood loss.

Restless legs syndrome. A neurological disease found in hemodialysis patients and involves an irresistible urge to move their legs.

Sleep apnea. A short cessation of breathing caused by blockage in the airways.

Sodium. A principal substance (salt) that determines how much fluid the body retains. Eating too much sodium can lead to high blood pressure.

Stem cells. Cells that develop shortly after the egg is fertilized but before they can become specialized cells of the body, such as kidney, heart, lung, or brain.

Tissue typing. *See* HLA typing.

Transplantation. Organ replacement therapy in which an organ from one individual, either living or deceased, is removed from a donor and placed in a recipient.

Urea. Breakdown product of protein. Urea is the main substance excreted by the kidney.

Uremia. Excess amount of urea in the blood, which can cause death in patients with kidney failure without dialysis or transplantation.

Uremic pruritis. Dry, itchy skin often seen in patients undergoing hemodialysis.

Ureters. Long tubes to connect the kidneys to the bladder.

Uric acid. A waste product of purines that can cause gout if in high concentrations in the blood.

Urinalysis. A method used to detect blood or protein in the urine. It can also be used to detect bacteria that may infect the kidney or bladder.

Urinary reduction rate (URR). A measure of efficiency in hemodialysis.

Vasopressin. A hormone released by the pituitary gland that acts on the kidney to retain fluid.

Vitamin D. A fat-soluble vitamin needed to form and maintain strong bones. Vitamin D can be made naturally or supplied in the diet or with supplements. The kidney makes the most active form of vitamin D, and when kidneys fail, bone structure can degrade, requiring treatment with the most active form. This problem is most common in hemodialysis patients.

Xenotransplantation. Transplantation of an organ from one species to another.

References

Chapter 1. Understanding Chronic Kidney Disease

1. A. S. Levi et al., "Nomenclature for kidney function and disease: report of a Kidney Disease: Improving Global Outcomes (KDIGO) Consensus Conference." *Kidney International* 97 (2020): 1117–1129.
2. M. Nagavi et al., "Global, regional, and national age–sex specific all-cause and cause-specific mortality for 240 causes of death, 1990–2013: A systematic analysis for the Global Burden of Disease Study 2013." *Lancet* 385 (2015): 117–171.
3. *United States Renal Data System: 2020 USRDS Annual Data Report; Epidemiology of Kidney Disease in the United States.* Bethesda, MD: National Institutes of Health, National Institute of Diabetes and Digestive and Kidney Diseases, 2020.
4. *United States Renal Data System: USRDS Annual Data Report; Epidemiology of Kidney Disease in the United States.* Bethesda, MD: National Institutes of Health, National Institute of Diabetes and Digestive and Kidney Diseases, 2018.
5. E. Kübler-Ross and D. Kessler, *On Grief and Grieving.* New York: Scribner, 2005.
6. M. Ford, *Caring for Renal Patients: A Caregiver's Guide to Chronic Kidney Disease; Information and Resources for Those Caring for Someone with CKD.* N.p.: Renal Diet HQ, 2017.

Chapter 3. Why Kidneys Fail

1. Obesity was measured by body mass index (BMI) weight in kilograms divided by the square of height in meters. A BMI greater than 25 is considered overweight, over 30 as obese, and over 40 as morbidly obese.
2. C. D. Fryer et al., *Prevalence of Overweight, Obesity, and Severe Obesity among Adults Aged 20 and Over: United States, 1960–1962 through 2015–2016* (NCHS Data Brief No 288). Hyattsville, MD: National Center for Health Statistics, 2018.
3. *Global Report on Diabetes.* Geneva: World Health Organization, 2016.
4. *Estimates of Diabetes and Its Burden in the United States, National Diabetes Statistics Report, 2017.* Atlanta, GA: Centers for Disease Control and Prevention, US Department of Human Services, 2020.
5. P. A. Diaz-Valencia et al., "Global epidemiology of type 1 diabetes in young adults and adults: A systematic review." *BMC Public Health* 15 (2015): 255.
6. R. A. Insel et al., "Staging presymptomatic type 1 diabetes: A scientific statement of JDRF, the Endocrine Society, and the American Diabetes Association." *Diabetes Care* 38 (2015): 1964–1974.

7. Y. Hu et al., "Antibiotics, gut microbiota, environment in early life and type 1 diabetes." *Pharmacological Reviews* 119 (2017): 219–226.

8. A. Katsarou et al., "Type 1 diabetes mellitus." *Nature Reviews Disease Primers* 3 (2017): 17016.

9. R. Respaut and C. Terhune, "U.S. insulin costs per patient nearly doubled from 2012 to 2016: Study." *Healthcare & Pharma*, January 22, 2019.

10. C. Ke et al., "Diabetes in the young: A population-based study of South Asian, Chinese and white people." *Diabetic Medicine* 32 (2015): 487–496.

11. J. I. Morton et al., "The association between age of onset of type 2 diabetes and the long-term risk of end-stage kidney disease: A national registry study." *Diabetes Care* 43 (2020): 1788–1795.

12. A. Stančáková and M. Laakso, "Genetics of type 2 diabetes." *Endocrine Reviews* 31 (2016): 203–220.

13. E. R. Pulgaron and A. M. Delmater, "Obesity and type 2 diabetes in children: Epidemiology and treatment." *Current Diabetes Reports* 14 (2014): 508.

14. W. Chen et al., "Hypothalamic insulin resistance in obesity: Effects on glucose homeostasis." *Neuroendocrinology* 104 (2017): 364–381.

15. S. Kullmann et al., "Intranasal insulin enhances brain functional connectivity mediating the relationship between adiposity and subjective feeling of hunger." *Scientific Reports* 7 (2017): 1627.

16. R. K. Singh et al., "Molecular genetics of human obesity: A comprehensive review." *Comptes Rendus Biologies* 340 (2017): 87–108.

17. D. Albuquerque et al., "Current review of genetics of human obesity: From molecular mechanisms to an evolutionary perspective." *Molecular Genetics and Genomics* 290 (2015): 1191–1121.

18. K. Aung et al., "Risk of developing diabetes and cardiovascular disease in metabolically unhealthy normal-weight and metabolically healthy obese individuals." *Journal of Clinical Endocrinology and Metabolism* 99 (2014): 462–468.

19. M. Roden and G. I. Shulman, "The integrative biology of type 2 diabetes." *Nature* 576 (2019): 51–60; N. Esser et al., "Inflammation as a link between obesity, metabolic syndrome and type 2 diabetes." *Diabetes Research and Clinical Practice* 105 (2014): 141–150.

20. X. Wei et al., "Fatty acid synthesis configures the plasma membrane for inflammation in diabetes." *Nature* 539 (2017): 294–298.

21. M. K. Salgaço et al., "Relationship between gut microbiota, probiotics, and type 2 diabetes mellitus." *Applied Microbiology and Biotechnology* 103 (2019): 9229–9238.

22. H. Liu et al., "Role of gut microbiota, bile acids and their cross-talk in the effects of bariatric surgery on obesity and type 2 diabetes." *Journal of Diabetes Investigation* 9 (2018): 13–20.

23. K. Tziomalos and V. G. Athyros, "Diabetic nephropathy: new risk factors and improvements in diagnosis." *Reviews of Diabetic Studies* 12 (2015): 110–118.

24. M. R. P. Karkus et al., "Prediabetes is associated with microalbuminuria, reduced kidney function and chronic kidney disease in the general popu-

lation: the KORA (Cooperative Health Research in the Augsburg Region) F4-Study." *Nutrition, Metabolism, and Cardiovascular Diseases* 28 (2018): 234–242.

25. E. J. Benjamin et al., "Heart disease and stroke statistics—2018 update: A report from the American Heart Association." *Circulation* 137 (2018): e67–e492.

26. P. Lloyd-Sherlock et al., "Hypertension among older adults in low- and middle-income countries: Prevalence, awareness, and control." *International Journal of Epidemiology* 43 (2014): 116–128.

27. M. W. Attaei et al., "Availability and affordability of blood pressure-lowering medicines and the effect on blood pressure control in high-income, middle-income, and low-income countries: an analysis of the PURE study data." *Lancet Public Health* 2 (2017): e411–e419.

28. P. K. Whelton et al., "2017 ACC/AHA/AAPA/ABC/ACPM/AGS/APhA/ASH/ ASPC/NMA/PCNA guideline for the prevention, detection, evaluation, and management of high blood pressure in adults." *Journal of the College of Cardiology* 71 (2018): e127–e248.

29. H. Ji et al., "Sex differences in blood pressure trajectories over the life course." *Journal of the American Medical Association Cardiology* 5 (2020): 19–26.

30. E. Evangelou et al., "Genetic analysis of over 1 million people identifies 535 new loci associated with blood pressure traits." *Nature Genetics* 50 (2018): 1412–1425; W. Manosroi and G. H. Williams, "Genetics of human primary hypertension: Focus on hormonal mechanisms." *Endocrine Reviews* 40 (2019): 825–856.

31. N. Musemwa and C. A. Gaegbeku, "Hypertension in African Americans." *Current Cardiology Reports* 19 (2017): 129.

32. E. Jones and B. Rayner, "The importance of the epithelial sodium channel in determining salt sensitivity in people of African origin." *Pediatric Nephrology* 36 (2021): 237–243.

33. D. K. Gupta et al., "Differences in natriuretic peptide levels by race/ethnicity (from the Multi-Ethnic Study of Atherosclerosis)." *American Journal of Cardiology* 120 (2017): 1008–1015.

34. A. Leiba et al., "Association of adolescent hypertension with future end-stage renal disease." *Journal of the American Medical Association Internal Medicine* 179 (2019): 517–523.

35. B. B. Bell and K. Rahmouni, "Leptin as a mediator of obesity-induced hypertension." *Current Obesity Reports* 5 (2016): 397–404.

36. M. Prager-Khoutorsky et al., "Role of vasopressin in rat models of salt-dependent hypertension." *Current Hypertension Reports* 19 (2017): 42.

37. P. Nakagawa and C. D. Sigmund, "How is the brain renin-angiotensin system regulated?" *Hypertension* 70 (2017): 10–18.

38. M. M. O'Shaughnessy et al., "Glomerular disease frequencies by race, sex and region: Results from the International Kidney Biopsy Survey." *Nephrology Dialysis Transplantation* 33 (2018): 661–669.

39. B. I. Freedman et al., "*APOL1*-associated nephropathy: a key contributor

to racial disparities in CKD." *American Journal of Kidney Diseases* 72 (2018, Suppl. 1): S8–S16.

40. A. Z. Rosenberg and J. B. Kopp, "Focal segmental glomerulosclerosis." *Clinical Journal of the American Society of Nephrology* 12 (2017): 502–517.
41. G. Stojan and M. Petri, "Epidemiology of systemic lupus erythematosus: An update." *Current Opinions in Rheumatology* 30 (2018): 144–150.
42. A. Javinani et al., "Exploring the etiopathogenesis of systemic lupus erythematosus: A genetic perspective." *Immunogenetics* 71 (2019): 283–297.
43. D. Azzouz et al., "Lupus nephritis is linked to disease-activity associated expansions and immunity to a gut commensal." *Annals of the Rheumatic Diseases* 78 (2019): 947–956.
44. C. Bergman et al., "Polycystic kidney disease." *Nature Review Disease Primers* 4 (2018): 50.
45. D. A. Maatje and V. E. Torres, "Polycystic kidney disease and the vasopressin pathway." *Annals of Nutrition and Metabolism* 70 Suppl.1 (2017): 43–50.
46. A. Alam et al., "Total kidney volume in autosomal dominant polycystic kidney disease: a biomarker of disease progression and therapeutic efficacy." *American Journal of Kidney Diseases* 66 (2015): 564–576.
47. R. W. Schrier et al., "Blood pressure in early autosomal dominant polycystic kidney disease." *New England Journal of Medicine* 371 (2014): 2255–2266.
48. I. M. Sanchis et al., "Presymptomatic screening for intracranial aneurysms in patients with autosomal dominant polycystic kidney disease." *American Journal of the American Society of Nephrology* 14 (2019): 1151–1160.
49. M. Baker and M. A. Perazella, "NSAIDs in CKD: Are they safe?" *American Journal of Kidney Diseases* 76 (2020): 546–557.
50. E. A. Hu et al., "Alcohol consumption and incident kidney disease: Results from the Atherosclerosis Risk in Communities Study." *Journal of Renal Nutrition* 30 (2020): 22–30.
51. H. He et al., "Alcohol consumption and incident diabetes: Results from the Atherosclerosis Risk in Communities (ARIC) Study." *Diabetologia* 62 (2019): 770–778.
52. J. L. Rein and C. M. Wyatt, "Marijuana and cannabinoids in ESRD and earlier CKD." *American Journal of Kidney Diseases* 71 (2018): 267–274.
53. B. Mills et al., "Synthetic cannabinoids." *American Journal of Medical Sciences* 350 (2015): 59–62.
54. R. J. Johnson et al., "Chronic kidney disease of unknown cause in agricultural communities." *New England Journal of Medicine* 380: 1843–1852.
55. M. B. Lanktree et al., "Evolving role of genetic testing for the clinical management of autosomal dominant polycystic kidney disease." *Nephrology Dialysis Transplantation* 34 (2019): 1453–1460.

Chapter 4. Diagnosing and Managing Chronic Kidney Disease

1. J. A. Vassalotti et al., "Practical approach to detection and management of chronic kidney disease for the primary care clinician," *American Journal of Medicine* 129 (2016): 153–162.

2. L. A. Inker et al., "KDOQI US commentary on the 2012 KDIGO Clinical Practice Guideline for the Evaluation and Management of CKD." *American Journal of Kidney Diseases* 63 (2014): 713–735.

3. S. U. Nigwekar et al., "Characterization and correction of olfactory deficits in kidney disease." *Journal of the American Society of Nephrology* 28 (2017): 3395–3403.

4. S. N. Davison et al., "Recommendations for the care of patients receiving conservative kidney management: Focus on management of CKD and symptoms." *Clinical Journal of the American Society of Nephrology* 14 (2019): 626–634.

5. "KIDIGO Clinical Practice Guideline for Anemia in Chronic Kidney Disease." *Kidney International Supplements* 2 (2012): 283–287.

6. M. Dobre et al., "Association of serum bicarbonate with risk of renal and cardiovascular outcomes in CKD: A report from the Chronic Renal Insufficiency Cohort (CRIC) study." *American Journal of Kidney Diseases* 62 (2013): 670–678.

7. G. N. Nakhoul et al., "Serum potassium, end-stage renal disease and mortality in chronic kidney disease." *American Journal of Nephrology* 41 (2015): 456–463.

8. A. J. Collins et al., "Association of serum potassium with all-cause mortality in patients with and without heart failure, chronic kidney disease, and/or diabetes." *American Journal of Nephrology* 46 (2017): 213–221.

9. S. P. Juraschek et al., "Association of kidney disease with prevalent gout in the United States in 1988–1994 and 2007–2010." *Seminars in Arthritis and Rheumatism* 42 (2013): 551–561.

10. J. A. Singh and J. D. Cleveland, "Gout is associated with a higher risk of chronic renal disease in older adults: A retrospective cohort of U.S. Medicare population." *BMC Nephrology* 20 (2019): 1–7.

11. A. B. Vargas-Santos et al., "Cause-specific mortality in gout: Novel findings of elevated risk of non-cardiovascular related deaths." *Arthritis and Rheumatology* 71 (2019): 1935–1942.

12. K. H. Yu, "Risk of end-stage renal disease associated with gout: A nationwide population study." *Arthritis Research & Therapy* 14 (2012): R83.

13. T. B. Bardin and P. Richette, "Impact of comorbidities on gout and hyperuricaemia: An update on prevalence and treatment options." *BMC Medicine* 15 (2017): 1–10.

14. A. B. Vargas-Santos and T. Meogi, "Management of gout and hyperuricemia in CKD." *American Journal of Kidney Diseases* 70 (2017): 422–439.

15. S. Palmer et al., "Prevalence of depression in chronic kidney disease: Systematic review and meta-analysis of observational studies." *Kidney International* 84 (2013): 179–191.

16. Y. C. Tsai et al., "Association of symptoms of depression with progression of CKD." *American Journal of Kidney Diseases* 60 (2012): 54–61.

17. N. G. Choi et al., "Financial barriers to health care access may increase distress in patients with CKD." *Kidney Medicine* 4 (2019): 162–170.

Chapter 5: Preventing, Postponing, and Treating Chronic Kidney Disease

1. K. H. Nam et al., "Carbohydrate-rich diet is associated with increased risk of incident chronic kidney disease in non-diabetic subjects." *Journal of Clinical Medicine* 8 (2019): 793.

2. I. Shai et al., "Weight loss with a low carbohydrate, Mediterranean, or low-fat diet." *New England Journal of Medicine* 359 (2008): 229–241.

3. *Guideline: Sugars intake for adults and children.* Geneva: World Health Organization, 2015.

4. *United States Renal Data System, 2020 Annual Data Report: Epidemiology of Kidney Disease in the United States.* Bethesda, MD: National Institutes of Health, National Institute of Diabetes and Digestive and Kidney Diseases, 2020.

5. L. Tellez et al., "Glucose utilization rates regulates intake levels of artificial sweeteners." *Journal of Physiology* 591 (2013): 5727–5744.

6. J. Lin and G. Curhan, "Associations of sugar and artificial sweetened soda with albuminuria and kidney function decline in women." *Clinical Journal of the American Society of Nephrology* 6 (2011): 160–166.

7. D. Swift et al., "The role of exercise and physical activity in weight loss and maintenance." *Progress in Cardiovascular Diseases* 56 (2014): 441–447.

8. H. MacKinnon et al., "The association of physical function and physical activity with all-cause mortality and adverse clinical outcomes in nondialysis chronic kidney disease: A systematic review." *Therapeutic Advances in Chronic Disease* 9 (2018): 209–226.

9. I. Chen et al., "Association of walking with survival and RRT among patients with CKD stages 3–5." *Clinical Journal of the American Society of Nephrology* 9 (2014): 1183–1189.

10. E. Howden et al., "Exercise training in CKD: Efficacy, adherence, and safety." *American Journal of Kidney Diseases* 65 (2015): 585–591.

11. D. Mozaffarian et al., "Global sodium consumption and death from cardiovascular causes." *New England Journal of Medicine* 14 (2014): 624–634.

12. E. McMahon et al., "A randomized trial of dietary sodium restriction in CKD." *Journal of the Society of Nephrology* 24 (2013): 2096–2103.

13. A. Drewnowski et al., "The feasibility of meeting the WHO guidelines for sodium and potassium: A cross-national comparison study." *BMJ Open* 5 (2015): e006625.

14. T. Kotchen et al., "Salt in health and disease—a delicate balance." *New England Journal of Medicine* 368 (2013): 1229–1237.

15. B. Riegel et al., "Patterns of adherence to diuretics, dietary sodium and fluid intake recommendations in adults with heart failure." *Heart and Lung: The Journal of Cardiopulmonary and Acute Care* 48 (2019): 179–185.

16. A. Spencer and P. Greasley, "Pharmacologic inhibition of intestinal sodium uptake: A gut centric approach to sodium management." *Current Opinions in Nephrology and Hypertension* 24 (2015): 410–416.

17. G. Ko et al., "Dietary protein intake and chronic kidney disease." *Current Opinion in Clinical Nutrition and Metabolic Care* 20 (2017): 77–85.

18. A. Noce et al., "Is low-protein diet a possible risk factor in malnutrition in chronic kidney disease patients?" *Cell Death Discovery* 2 (2016): 16026.

19. Y. Hou et al., "Phosphorus and mortality risk in end-stage renal disease: A meta-analysis." *Clinica Chimica Acta* 474 (2017): 108–113.

20. M. Calvo et al., "Dietary phosphate and the forgotten kidney patient: A critical need for FDA regulatory action." *American Journal of Kidney Diseases* 73 (2019): 542–551.

21. R. Feinman et al., "Dietary carbohydrate restriction as the first approach in diabetes management: Critical review and evidence base." *Nutrition* 31 (2015): 1–13.

22. E. Bekiari et al., "Artificial pancreas treatment for outpatients with type 1 diabetes: Systematic review and meta-analysis." *BMJ* 361 (2018): k1310.

23. C. Mathieu et al., "Insulin analogues in type 1 diabetes mellitus: Getting better all the time." *Nature Reviews Endocrinology* 13 (2017): 385–399.

24. D. Chou et al., "Glucose-responsive insulin activity by covalent modification with aliphatic phenylboronic acid conjugates." *Proceedings of the National Academy of Sciences* 112 (2015): 2401–2406.

25. J. Wang et al., "Glucose transporter inhibitor-conjugated insulin mitigates hypoglycemia." *Proceedings of the National Academy of Sciences* 116 (2019): 10744–10748.

26. F. Wittermayer et al., "Addressing unmet medical needs in type 1 diabetes: A review of drugs under development." *Current Diabetes Review* 13 (2017): 300–314.

27. A. Shapiro et al., "Clinical pancreatic islet transplantation." *Nature Reviews Endocrinology* 13 (2017): 268–277.

28. S. Zhu et al., "Human pancreatic beta-like cells converted from fibroblasts." *Nature Communications* 7 (2016): 10080.

29. J. Thrasher, "Pharmacologic management of type 2 diabetes mellitus: Available therapies." *American Journal of Cardiology* 120 (2017): S4–S16; C. Wanner et al., "Empagliflozin and clinical outcomes in patients with type 2 diabetes mellitus, established cardiovascular disease, and chronic kidney disease." *Circulation* 9 (2018): 119–129; V. Perkovic et al., "Canagliflozin and renal outcomes in type 2 diabetes and nephropathy." *New England Journal of Medicine* 380 (2019): 2295–2306.

30. Y. S. Lin et al., "Renal and glucose-lowering effects of empagliflozin and dapagliflozin in different chronic kidney disease stages." *Frontiers in Endocrinology* 10 (2019): 820; B. L. Neuen et al., "Relative and absolute risk reductions in cardiovascular and kidney outcomes with canagliflozin across KDIGO risk categories: Findings from the CANVAS Program." *American Journal of Kidney Diseases* 77 (2021): 23–34.e1; H. J. L. Heerspink et al., "Dapagliflozin in patients with chronic kidney disease." *New England Journal of Medicine* 383 (2020): 1436–1446.

31. A. Shah and B. Laferrère, "Diabetes after bariatric surgery." *Canadian Journal of Diabetes* 41 (2017): 401–406.

32. W. Garvey et al., "American Association of Clinical Endocrinologists and American College of Endocrinology comprehensive clinical practice guidelines for medical care of patients with obesity." *Endocrine Practice* 22 (2016): 1–205.

33. P. Georgianos and R. Agarwal, "Hypertension in chronic kidney disease: *Nephrology Dialysis Transplantation* notable 2017 advances." *Nephrology Dialysis Transplantation* 34 (2019): 1–4.

34. R. Furie et al., "Two-year, randomized, controlled trial of belimumab in lupus nephritis." *New England Journal of Medicine* 383 (2020): 1117–1128; B. H. Roven et al., "A randomized, controlled double-blind study comparing the efficacy and safety of dose-ranging voclosporin with placebo in achieving remission in patients with active lupus nephritis." *Kidney International* 95 (2019): 219–231; K. L. Gibson et al., "AURORA study: Voclosporin effective treatment for lupus nephritis." Abstract No. 407. Presented at National Kidney Foundation Spring Clinical Meetings, March 26–29, 2020.

35. M. van Gastel and V. Torres, "Polycystic kidney disease and the vasopressin pathway." *Annals of Nutrition and Metabolism* 70 (2017, Suppl. 1): 43–50.

Chapter 6. Dialysis

1. *U.S. Renal Data System, 2020 Annual Data Report: Atlas of End-Stage Renal Disease in the United States.* Bethesda, MD: National Institutes of Health, National Institute of Diabetes and Digestive and Kidney Diseases, 2020.

2. A. Niang et al., "Hemodialysis versus peritoneal dialysis in resource-limited settings." *Current Opinion in Nephrology and Transplantation* 27 (2018): 463–471; A. K. Bello et al., "Status of care for end stage kidney disease in countries and regions worldwide: International cross sectional survey." *BMJ* 367 (2019): l5873.

3. E. A. Brown, "Influence of reimbursement policies on dialysis modality distribution around the world." *Clinical Journal of the American Society of Nephrology* (2019): 10–12.

4. This description is the one that I employed when on peritoneal dialysis using supplies provided by Baxter International, Inc. Supplies from other companies, such as Fresenius, are also available.

5. S. Arya et al., "Sex and racial disparities in catheter use and dialysis access in the United States Medicare population." *Journal of the American Society of Nephrology* 31 (2020): 625–636.

6. B. Wong et al., "Buttonhole versus rope-ladder cannulation of arterio-venous graft for hemodialysis: A systematic study." *American Journal of Kidney Diseases* 64 (2014): 918–936.

7. S. Haroon and A. Davenport, "Choosing a dialyzer: What clinicians need to know." *Hemodialysis International* 22 (2018): S65–S74.

8. B. W. Miller et al., "Choosing home hemodialysis: a critical review of patient outcomes." *Blood Purification* 45 (2018): 224–229.

9. R. C. Walker et al., "Home hemodialysis: a comprehensive review of patient-centered and economic considerations." *Clinicoeconomics and Outcomes Research* 9 (2017): 149–161.

10. S. P. Y. Wong et al., "Care practices for patients with advanced kidney disease who forgo maintenance dialysis." *JAMA International Medicine* 179 (2019): 305–313.

11. M. W. Wachterman et al., "Framing prognostic expectations: One-year mortality after dialysis initiation among older adults." *JAMA Internal Medicine* 179 (2019): 987–990.

12. S. N. Davison et al., "Recommendations for the care of patients receiving conservative kidney management: Focus on management of CKD and symptoms." *Clinical Journal of the American Society of Nephrology* 14 (2019): 626–634.

13. J. S. Scherer et al., "Sleep disorders, restless legs syndrome, and uremic pruritis: Diagnosis and treatment of common symptoms in dialysis patients." *American Journal of Kidney Diseases* 69 (2017): 117–128.

14. C. H. Lin et al., "Obstructive sleep apnea and chronic kidney disease." *Current Opinions in Pulmonary Medicine* 24 (2018): 549–554.

15. H. Tominaga et al., "Association between bone mineral density, muscle volume, walking ability and geriatric nutritional risk index in hemodialysis patients." *Asia Pacific Journal of Clinical Nutrition* 27 (2018): 1062–1066.

16. S. C. Chen et al., "Associations among geriatric nutrition risk index, bone mineral density, body composition and handgrip strength in patients receiving hemodialysis." *Nutrition* 65 (2019): 6–12.

Chapter 7. Transplantation

1. W. R. Mulley et al., "Tissue typing for kidney transplantation for the general nephrologist." *Nephrology* 24 (2019): 997–1000.

2. A. K. Bello et al., "Status of care for end stage kidney disease in countries and regions worldwide: International cross sectional survey." *BMJ* 367 (2019): I5873; B. Mahillo et al., "Worldwide distribution of solid organ transplantation and access of populations to those practices." *Transplantation* 102 (2018): S71–S72.

3. A. K. Bello et al., "Assessment of global kidney health care status." *Journal of the American Medical Association* 317 (2017): 1864–1881.

4. J. D. Schold et al., "Effects of body mass index on kidney transplant outcomes are significantly modified by patient characteristics." *American Journal of Transplantation* 21, no. 2 (2020): 751–765.

5. C. Morath et al., "ABO-incompatible kidney transplantation." *Frontiers in Immunology* 8 (2017): 234.

6. This section is adapted from an article I wrote for the PKD Foundation, "Waiting for a kidney transplant." *PKD Progress* 18 (2003): 13.

7. N. Abrol et al., "Simultaneous bilateral laparoscopic nephrectomy with kidney transplantation in patients with ESRD due to ADPKD: A single-center experience." *American Journal of Transplantation* 21 (2021): 1513–1524.

8. J. E. Cooper, "Evaluation and treatment of acute rejection in kidney allografts." *Clinical Journal of the American Society of Nephrology* 15 (2020): 430–438.

9. D. E. Chute et al., "Direct-acting antiviral therapy for hepatitis C virus infection in the kidney transplant recipient." *Kidney International* 93 (2018): 560–567.

10. C. M. Durand et al., "Direct-acting antiviral prophylaxis in kidney transplantation from hepatitis C virus-infected donors to noninfected recipients: An open-label nonrandomized trial." *Annals of Internal Medicine* 168 (2018): 533–540.

Chapter 8. Future Treatment Options

1. E. Zeggini et al., "Translational genomics and precision medicine: Moving from the lab to the clinic." *Science* 365 (2019): 1409–1413.
2. D. A. Axelrod et al., "The impact of direct-acting antiviral agents on liver and kidney transplant costs and outcomes." *American Journal of Transplantation* 18 (2018): 2473–2482.
3. D. F. Reilly and M. D. Breyer, "The use of genomics to drive kidney disease drug discovery and development." *Clinical Journal of the American Society of Nephrology* 15 (2020): 1342–1351.
4. N. C. Baker et al., "A bibliometric review of drug repurposing." *Drug Discovery Today* 23 (2018): 661–672.
5. R. Barrangou and J. A. Doudna, "Applications of CRISPR technologies in research and beyond." *Nature Biotechnology* 34 (2018): 933–941.
6. N. W. Cruz and B. S. Freedman, "CRISPR gene editing in the kidney." *American Journal of Kidney Diseases* 71 (2018): 874–883.
7. A. V. Anzalone et al., "Search-and-replace genome editing without double stranded breaks or donor DNA." *Nature* 576 (2019): 149–157.
8. J. Siwy and H. Mischak, "Novel biological markers in kidney disease." *Kidney Update: Biomarkers for Kidney Disease*. Washington, DC: Science/AAAS, 2019, pp. 4–8.
9. C. Pontillo et al., "Prediction of chronic kidney disease stage 3 by CKD273, a urinary proteomic biomarker." *Kidney International Reports* 2 (2017): 1066–1075.
10. A. S. Klinger, "More intensive hemodialysis." *Clinical Journal of the American Society of Nephrology* 4 (2009): S121–S124.
11. M. Salani et al., "Innovations in wearable and implantable artificial kidneys." *American Journal of Kidney Diseases* 72 (2018): 745–751.
12. J. A. Bluestone and M. Anderson, "Tolerance in the age of immunity." *New England Journal of Medicine* 383 (2020): 1156–1166.
13. J. M. Mathew and J. R. Leventhal, editors, "Clinical transplant tolerance." *Human Immunology* 79 (2018): 255–402.
14. T. E. Wijkstrom et al., "Renal xenotransplantation: Experimental progress and clinical prospects." *Kidney International* 91 (2017): 790–796.
15. L. A. Padilla et al., "Attitudes to clinical pig kidney xenotransplantation among medical providers and patients." *Kidney 360* (2020): 657–662.
16. J. Marcheque et al., "Concise reviews: stem cells and kidney regeneration: An update." *Stem Cells Translational Medicine* 8 (2019): 82–92.
17. K. Hariharan et al., "Assembling kidney tissues from cells: The long road from organoids to organs." *Frontiers in Cell and Developmental Biology* 3 (2015): 70; T. Takebe and J. W. Wells, "Organoids by design." *Science* 364 (2019): 956–959.

18. S. Park et al., "Organoids-on-a-chip." *Science* 364 (2019): 960–965.
19. K. A. Horman et al., "Flow-enhanced vascularization and maturation of kidney organoids in vitro." *Nature Methods* 16 (2019): 255–262.
20. S. Pondrom, "3D printing in transplantation." *American Journal of Transplantation* 16 (2016): 1339–1340.
21. A. Do et al., "3D printing of scaffolds for tissue regeneration applications." *Advances in Healthcare Materials* 4 (2015): 1741–1762.

Appendix

1. M. Nagavi et al., "Global, regional, and national age–sex specific all-cause and cause-specific mortality for 240 causes of death, 1990–2013: A systematic analysis for the Global Burden of Disease Study 2013." *Lancet* 385 (2015): 117–171.
2. *United States Renal Data System: 2020 Annual Data Report; Epidemiology of Kidney Disease in the United States.* Bethesda, MD: National Institutes of Health, National Institute of Diabetes and Digestive and Kidney Diseases, 2020.
3. CORR Annual Statistics: Renal replacement therapy (dialysis and transplantation) for ESKD, 2007 to 2016 (2017). corr_ar-kidney-data-tables-en .xlsx.
4. M. Gonzalez-Bedat et al., "Burden of disease: prevalence and incidence of ESRD in Latin America." *Clinical Nephrology* 83 (2015, Suppl. 1): 3–6.
5. A. Kramer et al., "The European Renal Association—European Dialysis and Transplant Association (ERA—EDTA) Registry Annual Report 2016: A summary." *Clinical Kidney Journal* (2019): 1–19.
6. S. Abd ElHafeez et al., "Prevalence and burden of chronic kidney disease among the general population and high-risk groups in Africa: A systematic review." *BMJ Open* 8 (2018): 1–32.
7. Y. Farag et al., "Chronic kidney disease in the Arab world: A call for action." *Nephron Clinical Practice* 121 (2012): c120–c123.
8. F. Shaheen et al., "Preventative strategies of renal failure in the Arab world." *Kidney International* 68 (2005, Suppl.): S37–S40.
9. A. Dare et al., "Renal failure deaths and their risk factors in India 2001–13: Nationally representative estimates from the Million Death Study." *Lancet* 5 (2017): e89–e95.
10. L. Zhang et al., "Prevalence of chronic kidney disease in China: A cross-sectional survey." *Lancet* 379 (2012): 815–822.
11. ANZDATA Registry, 40th Report, Australia and New Zealand Dialysis and Transplant Registry. Adelaide, Australia. 2017.
12. W. Hoy et al., "An expanded nationwide view of chronic kidney disease in Aboriginal Australians." *Nephrology* 21 (2016): 916–922.

Resources

1. K. Singh et al., "Patients' and nephrologists' evaluation of patient-facing smartphone apps for CKD." *Clinical Journal of the American Society of Nephrology* 14 (2019): 523–529.

Index

About the Author

Walter Hunt, PhD, holds a bachelor's degree in chemistry from Bethany College and a doctorate in neuropharmacology from West Virginia University. As a medical researcher for forty years, he examined the biological basis of diseases never considering that one day he would have to deal with a serious disease of his own. Having polycystic kidney disease (PKD), the fourth leading cause of kidney failure, he suffered seven and half years of dialysis and two dozen stays in the hospital before receiving the gift of life of a transplant. Dr. Hunt is also the author of *Writing My Name in the Snow: How I Adapted to Kidney Failure, Found My Inner Strength, and Began Life Anew* and he formerly served on the Board of Trustees of the PKD Foundation. Now free of kidney problems, Dr. Hunt travels the world.